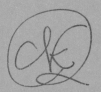

101

—BEST—

GLUTEN-FREE FOODS

pil

Publications International, Ltd.

Photography on pages 9, 21, 41, 85 and 103 by
PIL Photo Studio, Chicago.
Photographer: Justin Paris
Photographer's Assistant: Annemarie Zelasko
Food Stylists: Amy Andrews, Carol Smoler
Assistant Food Stylists: Lissa Levy, Breanna Moeller

All recipes and recipe photographs copyright
© Publications International, Ltd.

Recipe development on pages 9, 41 and 103
by Carol Emory.

Recipe development on pages 9, 21, 39 and 85
by Allison S. Kahen, RD, LDN.

Contributing writers: Carol Emory and Allison S.
Kahen, RD, LDN.

Recipes pictured on the front cover: Stuffed Squash
with Black Beans *(page 7)* and Gluten-Free Apple Pie
(page 71).
Recipe pictured on the back cover: Vietnamese
Summer Rolls *(page 145)*.

Photo Credits

Front Cover: Shutterstock

Back Cover: Thinkstock

Interior Art: Thinkstock and Shutterstock

ISBN-13: 978-1-4508-5126-8
ISBN-10: 1-4508-5126-6

Library of Congress Control Number: 2012934415

Manufactured in China.

8 7 6 5 4 3 2 1

Nutritional Analysis: Every effort has been made to
check the accuracy of the nutritional information that
appears with each recipe. However, because numerous
variables account for a wide range of values for
certain foods, nutritive analyses in this book should
be considered approximate. Different results may be
obtained by using different nutrient databases and
different brand-name products.

Microwave Cooking: Microwave ovens vary in
wattage. Use the cooking times as guidelines and
check for doneness before adding more time.

Note: This publication is only intended to provide
general information. The information is specifically
not intended to be a substitute for medical diagnosis
or treatment by your physician or other health care
professional. You should always consult your own
physician or other health care professionals about
any medical questions, diagnosis, or treatment.
(Products vary among manufacturers. Please check
labels carefully to confirm that the products you use
are free of gluten.) **Not all recipes in this book are
appropriate for all people with celiac disease,
gluten intolerance, food allergies or sensitivities.**

The information obtained by you from this book
should not be relied upon for any personal, nutritional,
or medical decision. You should consult an appropriate
professional for specific advice tailored to your specific
situation. PIL makes no representations or warranties,
express or implied, with respect to your use of this
information.

In no event shall PIL, its affiliates or advertisers be
liable for any direct, indirect, punitive, incidental,
special, or consequential damages, or any damages
whatsoever including, without limitation, damages for
personal injury, death, damage to property, or loss of
profits, arising out of or in any way connected with
the use of any of the above-referenced information or
otherwise arising out of the use of this book.

Publications International, Ltd.

What Is Gluten?

Gluten is a protein that is found in wheat, rye and barley. There are many reasons people avoid gluten. Some people are allergic to wheat itself while others may have a sensitivity to gluten and just feel better when they avoid it. The most serious is Celiac Disease, in which the body produces an autoimmune response after eating gluten. The only way to manage this condition is to follow a strict gluten-free diet.

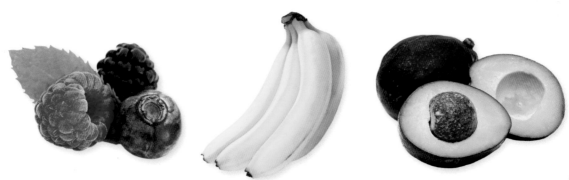

No More Bread? No Pasta?

At first, going gluten-free may appear to be rather limiting. Fortunately, there are many more delicious foods on the gluten-free list than on the forbidden list. There are also more and more products, from cereals to baking mixes to pastas, which are now being formulated in gluten-free versions. These days you'll find them not just in health food stores and online, but also on the shelves of most major supermarkets.

Some Good News

Spotting hidden gluten in processed foods is a lot easier now thanks to the FDA's Food Allergy Labeling Law that went into effect in 2004. Since wheat is a common allergen, any product that contains wheat or is derived from it must say so on the label. That means formerly questionable ingredients, such as modified food starch or maltodextrin, must now show wheat as part of their name if they were made from it (for example, "wheat maltodextrin"). Be aware that this ONLY applies to foods produced in the US and Canada. Imports are a different matter.

More Good News

Look at your dietary restrictions as an opportunity to try new foods. Add quinoa and chickpea flour to your cupboard. Use corn tortillas to make sandwiches or lasagna. You'll find easy recipes in this cookbook that are so delicious you'll forget that they're gluten-free. Healthy eating may actually be easier without gluten, too. Adding more fresh produce to your meals, eating less processed food and avoiding refined flour are all steps to a better diet for anyone.

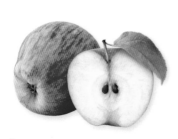
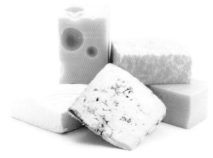
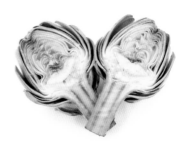

Gluten-Free Flour Blends

While there are many products that are now readily available in the supermarkets, they can be rather expensive. We have provided two basic flour blends that can be prepared in bulk and kept on hand for use at any time. Please refer to these when preparing many of the recipes in this cookbook.

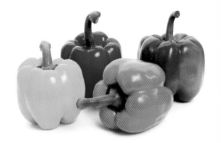

gluten-free all-purpose flour blend

    1 cup white rice flour
    1 cup sorghum flour
    1 cup tapioca flour
    1 cup cornstarch
    1 cup almond flour or coconut flour

Combine all ingredients in large bowl. Whisk to make sure flours are evenly distributed. The recipe can be doubled or tripled. Store in airtight container in refrigerator.

Makes about 5 cups

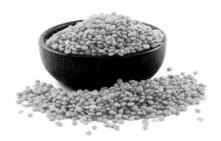

gluten-free flour blend for breads

    1 cup brown rice flour
    1 cup sorghum flour
    1 cup tapioca flour
    1 cup cornstarch
    ¾ cup millet flour*
    ⅓ cup instant mashed potato flakes

*If millet flour is not available substitute chickpea flour.

Combine all ingredients in large bowl. Whisk to make sure ingredients are evenly distributed. The recipe can be doubled or tripled. Store in airtight container in refrigerator.

Makes about 5 cups

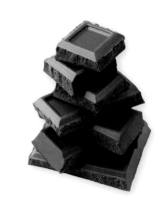

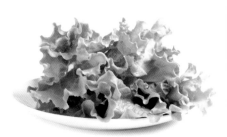

Acorn Squash

For people on a gluten-free diet, this acorn-shaped variety of winter squash is a star. It's simple to prepare and full of flavor and nutrients.

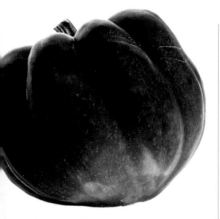

Benefits

Acorn squash is filled with important nutrients that are commonly lacking in a gluten-free diet because they're found in many gluten-containing foods. It is high in fiber, nearly 5 grams in a mere ½ cup serving, which is pertinent for people on gluten-free diets because it helps to keep their digestive systems healthy. Acorn squash is rich in two other important nutrients for people who don't eat gluten— vitamin B_6 and folate—both of which are often found added to gluten-containing processed foods like breads and cereals. Acorn squash is also rich in vitamins A and C and the mineral potassium.

Selection and Storage

You may find acorn squash year-round, but it's best from early fall to late winter. Look for acorn squash that is deeply colored (dark green with some golden coloring) and free of spots, bruises and mold. The hard skin serves as a barrier, allowing it to be stored a month or more in a cool, dark place.

Preparation

Acorn squash can be baked, steamed, sautéed, simmered or microwaved. One of the easiest ways to prepare an acorn squash is to cut one in half, scoop out the seeds and bake at 400°F for about 45 minutes. It may be difficult to cut raw, due to the tough, thick skin. To make cutting easier, soften squash in the microwave. Pierce the skin with a fork and microwave on HIGH for 1 to 2 minutes. Let the squash stand a few minutes to cool slightly before cutting. Then, simply slice lengthwise and remove the seeds.

Recipe Suggestions

Enjoy acorn squash as a side dish or make a filled half of acorn squash the center of your meal. You can serve the baked squash in the skin and fill the center with whatever you like (try rice, veggies and garlic), or you can scoop out the baked flesh and enjoy it mashed and sprinkled with a small amount of Parmesan cheese or other seasonings. Acorn squash is also a tasty addition to savory stews or soups. The creamy texture gives soups a hearty, thick consistency.

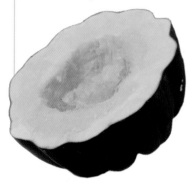

stuffed squash with black beans

1 cup water, divided
1 acorn squash (2 pounds),
    quartered, seeded, skin pierced
    with fork
Salt and black pepper
⅓ cup pine nuts (1½ ounces)
Nonstick cooking spray
1 cup chopped onion
1 medium red bell pepper, chopped
1 teaspoon ground cinnamon
¼ teaspoon ground allspice (optional)
1 cup canned black beans, rinsed
    and drained
¼ cup raisins
1 teaspoon sugar (optional)
¼ teaspoon salt
2 ounces crumbled goat cheese or
    feta cheese (optional)

1. Place ½ cup water in 8-inch square microwavable dish. Place squash, skin side up, in dish. Sprinkle with salt and black pepper. Cover with plastic wrap. Microwave on HIGH 12 minutes or until tender.

2. Meanwhile, heat medium nonstick skillet over medium-high heat. Add pine nuts; cook and stir 1 minute or until lightly browned. Remove to plate.

3. Spray skillet with cooking spray. Add onion and bell pepper; spray with cooking spray. Cook and stir 5 minutes or until vegetables just begin to brown. Add cinnamon and allspice, if desired; cook and stir 30 seconds. Add beans, raisins, sugar, if desired, and ¼ teaspoon salt. Stir in remaining ½ cup water. Remove from heat. Cover; let stand 2 minutes.

4. Spoon bean mixture into center of each squash piece. Sprinkle with pine nuts and cheese, if desired.

Makes 4 servings

nutrients per serving:

Calories 223	**Total Fat** 8g
Calories from Fat 35%	**Saturated Fat** 1g
Protein 6g	**Cholesterol** 0mg
Carbohydrate 39g	**Sodium** 356mg
Fiber 7g	

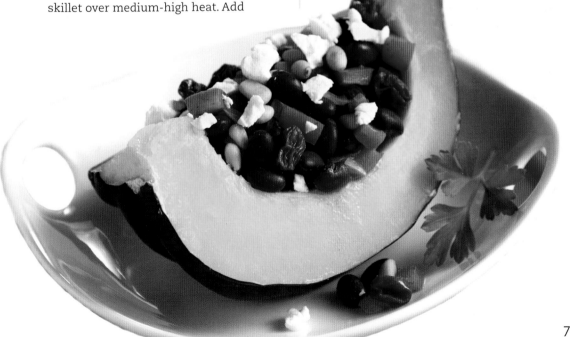

Almonds

Although we call them nuts, almonds are actually the seeds of the fruit from an almond tree. We don't eat the outer fruit, just the flavorful and nutrient-rich seeds.

Benefits

Almonds pack a powerful nutrient punch in a small package. Their combination of protein, fiber and healthy fats makes them a great food that provides lasting energy. They also contain vitamin E, magnesium, calcium and B vitamins. For people on a gluten-free diet, almonds serve as a great substitute for many wheat-containing ingredients, such as replacing crunchy croutons in salads. When finely ground, they work well as a coating for fish or chicken instead of bread crumbs.

Selection and Storage

Almonds are available packaged or in bulk, with or without shells. Packaged almonds are available in various forms—whole, blanched (with the skins removed), sliced, slivered, raw, dry- or oil-roasted, smoked, flavored and salted or unsalted. If purchasing flavored almonds, check the ingredient list and label to be sure they are free of gluten. Almonds in the shell can keep for a few months in a cool, dry location. Once you shell them or open a package of nuts, they will need to be stored in the refrigerator or freezer.

Preparation

Almonds can be used in many ways, but toasting almonds before using them really brings out their flavor. To toast almonds in the oven, spread them in a single layer on a baking sheet and bake at 350°F for 5 to 7 minutes or until they are golden brown, stirring occasionally. You may also toast them on the stove: Spread almonds in a single layer in a heavy-bottomed skillet and cook over medium heat 1 to 2 minutes or until the nuts are lightly browned, stirring frequently. Be sure to cool toasted nuts before using in recipes.

Recipe Suggestions

Almonds make a great snack on their own, or you can make your own trail mix and combine them with other nuts, gluten-free cereals, dried fruits and chocolate. Almonds make a great crunchy topping on salads, soups, casseroles, vegetable dishes, stir-fries, desserts and more. To use as a substitute for bread crumbs, place the almonds in a food processor and pulse until they are finely ground. Combine the ground nuts with herbs and spices that complement the flavors of the dish you are preparing.

banana-coconut cream pie

Crust

- 1 cup almonds
- 1 tablespoon sugar
- ½ cup flaked coconut
- ¼ cup (½ stick) butter, cut into pieces
- Pinch salt

Filling

- 2 bananas
- 1 teaspoon lemon juice
- ½ cup sugar
- ¼ cup cornstarch
- ¼ teaspoon salt
- 3 cups whole milk
- 2 egg yolks
- 1 teaspoon vanilla

Topping

- 1 banana
- 2 tablespoons flaked coconut
- Whipped cream

1. Preheat oven to 350°F. Grease 9-inch pie pan.

2. Place almonds and 1 tablespoon sugar in food processor; process using on/off pulsing action until almonds are ground. Add ½ cup coconut; pulse to combine. Add butter and pinch of salt; pulse until mixture begins to stick together. Pour into prepared pie pan; press onto bottom and up side. Bake 10 to 12 minutes or until golden around edge. Cool completely.

3. Slice 2 bananas; sprinkle with lemon juice. Layer on bottom of prepared crust.

4. Combine ½ cup sugar, cornstarch and ¼ teaspoon salt in medium saucepan. Whisk milk and egg yolks in medium bowl until well blended; slowly stir into sugar mixture. Cook and stir over medium heat until thickened. Bring to a boil; boil 1 minute. Remove from heat; stir in vanilla.

5. Pour mixture into crust over bananas. Cover and refrigerate at least 2 hours or until ready to serve.

6. Slice remaining banana; arrange on top of pie. Sprinkle with 2 tablespoons coconut and top with dollops of whipped cream. *Makes 8 servings*

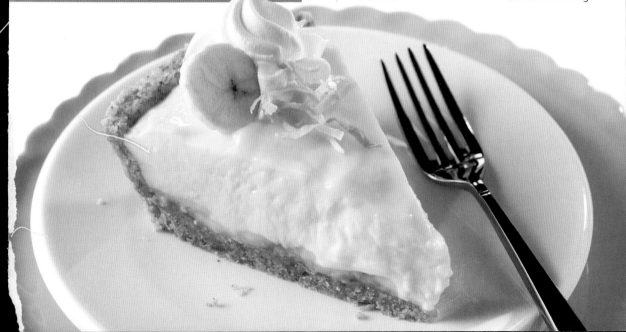

Almond Flour

Because almond flour works so well in baking, it is a staple in any gluten-free kitchen. Although it may be pricey, the results from using it make it worth it.

Benefits

Almond flour has a sweet, nutty taste and moistness that add flavor and texture to breads, muffins, cakes, cookies and other desserts. It has lower carbohydrate and higher protein contents than many other wheat-free flours. It isn't only used in gluten-free baking; its wonderful profile has made it a traditional ingredient in classic French desserts and Passover cooking.

Selection and Storage

Almond flour, also called almond powder and almond meal, is available at natural food stores and in the specialty flour section at many supermarkets or may be ordered online. It comes in two forms, blanched and unblanched. Blanched almond flour—or almond powder—is often used and is made from almonds that have had their skins removed, giving it a lighter color than unblanched almond flour, which is also called almond meal. Blanched almond flour has a finer texture, which is why it is preferred over unblanched almond flour. If purchasing almond flour in bulk quantities, it is best to freeze it and keep a small amount in the refrigerator.

Preparation

You can make your own almond flour by pulverizing blanched almonds in a food processor. It is very easy to end up with almond butter, so beware! Almond flour can be used in baking on its own, but for many recipes, it works well when combined with other wheat-free flours. It is a key component in the all-purpose flour blend that is referenced in many of the recipes in this book.

Recipe Suggestions

The most popular dessert using almond flour is the petite French pastry, the macaron. Macarons are crisp, yet chewy sandwich cookies filled with any desired filling, typically a flavored frosting or fruit jam. The base of the cookie is made from almond flour, egg whites, powdered and granulated sugars. It is often confused with the more popular coconut macaroon, which uses coconut instead of almond flour. Almond flour is also used in another French dish, clafouti, a baked dish that is made by topping fresh fruit with a custard-like batter. A traditional clafouti is made with cherries, but berries, plums, peaches and pears can be used.

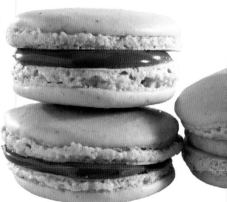

pistachio macarons

- ⅓ cup unsalted shelled pistachios (1½ ounces)
- 1½ cups powdered sugar
- ⅔ cup blanched almond flour
- 3 egg whites, at room temperature*
- 2 or 3 drops green food coloring
- ¼ cup granulated sugar
- Chocolate Ganache (recipe follows)

For best results, separate the eggs while cold. Leave the egg whites at room temperature for 3 or 4 hours. Reserve yolks in refrigerator for another use.

1. Line baking sheets with parchment paper. Double baking sheets by placing another sheet underneath each to protect macarons from burning or cracking. (Do not use insulated baking sheets.)

2. Place pistachios in food processor; pulse about 1 minute or until coarsely ground. Add powdered sugar and almond flour; pulse 2 to 3 minutes or until well combined into very fine powder, scraping bowl occasionally. Sift mixture twice; discard any remaining large pieces.

3. Beat egg whites in large bowl with electric mixer at high speed until foamy. Add food coloring. Gradually add granulated sugar; beat at high speed 2 to 3 minutes or until stiff, shiny peaks form, scraping bowl occasionally.

4. Add half of sifted pistachio mixture to egg whites. Stir with spatula to combine (about 12 strokes). Repeat with remaining pistachio mixture. Mix 15 strokes more by pressing against side of bowl and scooping from bottom until batter is smooth and shiny. (Check consistency by dropping spoonful of batter onto plate. It should have a peak which quickly relaxes back into batter. Do not overmix or undermix.)

5. Attach ½-inch plain piping tip to pastry bag. Scoop batter into bag. Pipe 1-inch circles about 2 inches apart onto prepared baking sheets. Tap baking sheets on flat surface to remove air bubbles. Let rest, uncovered, until tops harden slightly, about 15 minutes on dry days to 1 hour in more humid conditions. Gently touch top of macaron to check. When batter does not stick, macarons are ready to bake.

6. Meanwhile, preheat oven to 375°F.** Place oven rack in center. Place one sheet of macarons in oven. Bake 5 minutes. *Reduce oven temperature to 325°F.* Bake 10 to 13 minutes, checking at 5 minute intervals. (If macarons begin to brown, cover loosely with foil and reduce oven temperature or prop oven door open slightly with wooden spoon.) Repeat with remaining baking sheet.

7. Cool completely on pan on wire rack. While cooling, if they appear to be sticking to parchment, lift parchment edges and spray pan underneath lightly with water. (Steam will help release macarons.)

8. Meanwhile, prepare Chocolate Ganache. When macarons are completely cool, match same size cookies; spread bottom macaron with ganache and top with another. Store macarons in covered container in refrigerator up to five days. Freeze for longer storage.

Makes 16 to 20 macarons (1 macaron per serving)

**Oven temperature is crucial. Use an oven thermometer, if possible.*

Chocolate Ganache: Place 4 ounces chopped semisweet or bittersweet chocolate in shallow bowl. Heat ½ cup whipping cream in small saucepan over low heat until bubbles form around edge. Pour cream over chocolate; let stand 5 minutes. Stir until smooth.

Variation: For pistachio filling, combine 1 cup powdered sugar and ⅓ cup pistachios in food processor; process 2 to 3 minutes or until coarse paste forms, scraping bowl occasionally. Add 6 tablespoons softened butter and ½ teaspoon vanilla; pulse to combine.

nutrients per serving:

Calories 155	**Total Fat** 9g
Calories from Fat 47%	**Saturated Fat** 3g
Protein 3g	**Cholesterol** 10mg
Carbohydrate 19g	**Sodium** 13mg
Fiber 1g	

Amaranth

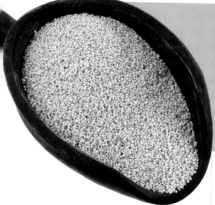

Amaranth is an ancient whole grain that is full of nutrients. Once a staple in the Aztec diet, this tiny Mexican-cultivated seed should be enjoyed in modern times in a gluten-free diet.

Benefits

Amaranth is high in fiber and protein. Even more, it contains a large amount of high-quality protein that isn't present in other grains. It is also a good source of iron and vitamin C. Where it deserves to be recognized is as a calcium source, providing nearly four times more calcium than wheat does.

Selection and Storage

You can find amaranth seeds at the supermarket with other grains or in bulk bins at natural food stores. It can also be found in other forms, including as cereal, in both puffed and flaked forms, or ground for use as gluten-free flour. It is most commonly found as the traditional Mexican candy called Alegría, a popped amaranth sticky candy bar.

Preparation

Amaranth is very easy to prepare. Combine it with water or any other desired liquid, such as chicken or vegetable broth, in a saucepan. About 1 cup of dried amaranth will require 2½ to 3 cups of liquid. Bring the amaranth and liquid to a boil over high heat. Reduce heat and simmer until all of the liquid is absorbed, about 20 minutes. Then, rinse the amaranth under cold running water. It is important that a fine-mesh strainer is used for rinsing, as these small grains will slide through the holes of a traditional strainer. Amaranth seeds can also be prepared like popcorn on a stovetop. Just cook the seeds in a skillet over high heat, stirring constantly until they pop.

Recipe Suggestions

Amaranth's nutty flavor and texture works well as a substitute for many rice or quinoa dishes. Try serving it cold with mixed vegetables in a salad, or warm as a stuffing for bell peppers or tomatoes. It also can be combined with other gluten-free grains for a nutritious side dish. Or get creative and try making your own snack mixes or snack bars using popped amaranth seeds.

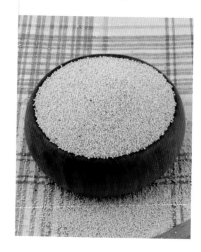

No-Bake Fruit 'n' Grain Bars

½ **cup uncooked amaranth**
2 **cups gluten-free whole grain puffed rice cereal**
½ **cup chopped dried fruits**
½ **cup honey**
½ **cup sugar**
¾ **cup almond butter**

1. Spray 8- or 9-inch square baking pan with nonstick cooking spray.

2. Heat medium saucepan over high heat. Add 1 tablespoon amaranth; stir or gently shake saucepan until almost all seeds have popped. (Partially cover saucepan if seeds are popping over the side.) Remove to medium bowl. Repeat with remaining amaranth.

3. Stir cereal and dried fruits into popped amaranth.

4. Combine honey and sugar in same saucepan; bring just to a boil over medium heat. Remove from heat; stir in almond butter until smooth.

5. Pour honey mixture over cereal mixture; stir until evenly coated. Press firmly into prepared pan. Let stand until set. Cut into bars.

Makes 16 bars

nutrients per serving:

Calories 145
Calories from Fat 43%
Protein 2g
Carbohydrate 20g
Fiber 1g
Total Fat 7g
Saturated Fat 1g
Cholesterol 0mg
Sodium 59mg

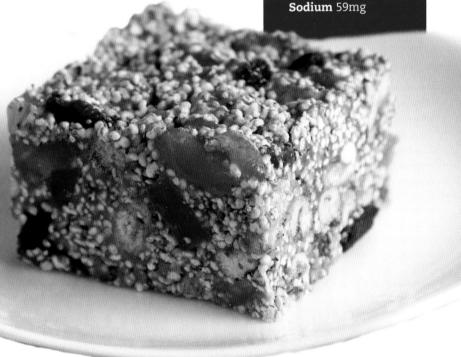

Apples

There are thousands of apple varieties grown today and new types being created each year. Whether you prefer tart or sweet, crisp and crunchy or soft and juicy, apples make a great food in any diet.

Benefits

Apples' versatility and nutrient content make them an excellent food to incorporate into your diet. Their crispness makes them a satisfying snack or salad topper, and their delightful flavor and high moisture content are what make them great for baking. They are filled with important nutrients too, including vitamin C and soluble fiber. The soluble fiber is what makes apples an excellent snack by filling us up.

Selection and Storage

Apples are at their peak—with maximum flavor and texture—from September through November.

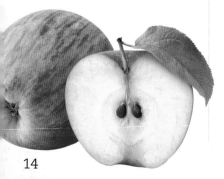

Choose apples that are firm and bright in color. The skin should be without any bruises, blemishes or punctures. Apples prefer humid air, so store them in the crisper drawer of the refrigerator. Some varieties will keep for several months, though most get mealy within a month.

Preparation

Choose apples for their intended purpose. A few varieties, like Golden Delicious, Granny Smith and Winesap, are all-purpose apples. For baking, try Empire, Rome Beauty, Cortland, Northern Spy or Ida Red; they keep their shape when cooked. Other popular varieties, including Red Delicious, Jonathan and McIntosh, are best eaten raw because they can lose their flavor and shape when cooked. Always wash your apples. Supermarket apples are often waxed to lock in moisture, but the wax also seals in pesticide residues on the skins. Peeling apples will remove the film but also a lot of the fiber. Just rinse apples under warm water to remove the wax. To prevent browning when cutting apples, sprinkle some lemon juice on cut surfaces.

Recipe Suggestions

Apples work well in many gluten-free dishes, from sweet to savory. They are often used in breakfast dishes and desserts but provide a ton of flavor and texture when incorporated into stuffing, rice or vegetable side dishes. You can add sautéed apples to virtually any dish. Cook and stir diced apples in melted butter with cinnamon in a small skillet. Be sure to keep the peel on to get all of the nutrients. Top your morning bowl of hot cereal with sautéed apples or combine them with some sliced carrots or other crunchy veggies.

spicy apple butter

5 pounds tart cooking apples (McIntosh, Granny Smith, Rome Beauty or York Imperial), peeled, cored and quartered (about 10 large apples)
1 cup sugar
½ cup apple juice
2 teaspoons ground cinnamon
½ teaspoon ground cloves
½ teaspoon ground allspice

Slow Cooker Directions

1. Combine all ingredients in slow cooker. Cover; cook on LOW 8 to 10 hours or until apples are very tender.

2. Mash apples with potato masher. Cook, uncovered, on LOW 2 hours or until thickened, stirring occasionally to prevent sticking.   *Makes about 6 cups (2 tablespoons per serving)*

Serving Suggestion: Spread apple butter on your favorite gluten-free bread or muffin.

nutrients per serving:

Calories 20	**Total Fat** 0g
Calories from Fat 0%	**Saturated Fat** 0g
Protein 0g	**Cholesterol** 0mg
Carbohydrate 5g	**Sodium** 0mg
Fiber 1g	

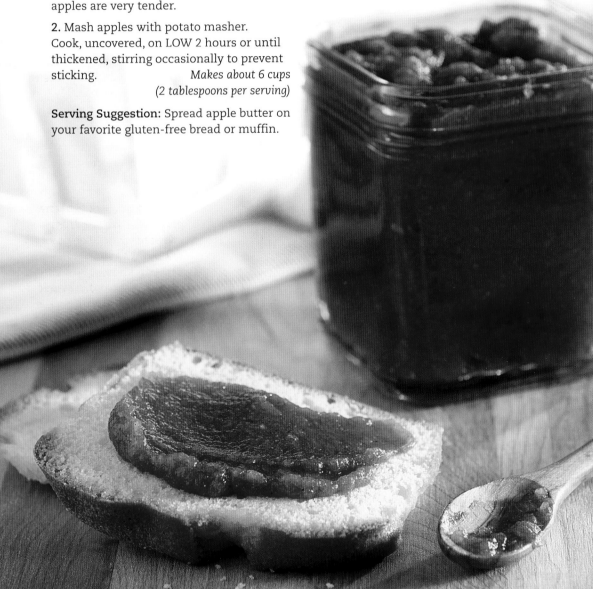

Applesauce

This childhood favorite goes above and beyond its typical use as a snack when used in baking. While applesauce is commonly used in low-fat and diabetic baking, its benefits make it great for a gluten-free diet, too.

Benefits

The sweet flavor, smooth texture and high moisture content of applesauce are what make it such a versatile ingredient and a must-have food in your pantry. It has been used as a replacement for butter and oil in low-fat baking for years—which makes it a plus for anyone who is not only allergic to gluten but also to dairy. If you choose to replace the oil in a recipe with applesauce, use about half the amount of applesauce as the oil is called for. For those who need or choose to avoid eggs, applesauce is a good substitute, as it binds ingredients the way eggs do. Applesauce is used in diabetic recipes because it is a great way to reduce the amount of added sugar in baked goods. And its mild flavor and natural sweetness make it an excellent way to incorporate fruit into the diet of picky eaters.

Selection and Storage

Applesauce is readily available at the supermarket and now comes in a variety of flavors. Be sure to read labels to be sure no gluten-containing flavoring or additives are listed. Generally, unsweetened applesauce works best in baking.

Preparation

Try making your own applesauce. You can use almost any type of apple, but McIntosh, Jonathan and Rome Beauty apples work best. Depending on the variety, the results will vary in sweetness and texture. To make about 5 cups of applesauce, combine 10 peeled and cored apples, ¾ cup packed brown sugar, ½ cup apple juice or cider, 1½ teaspoons ground cinnamon, ⅛ teaspoon ground nutmeg and ⅛ teaspoon salt in a large saucepan. Cover and cook over medium-low heat for 40 to 45 minutes or until the apples are tender, stirring occasionally to break up any chunks. Remove from heat and cool completely. For a smoother texture, place the mixture in a food processor or blender and process until the desired consistency is reached.

Recipe Suggestions

Using applesauce in baking works best with fruity flavored desserts, especially ones with spices like cinnamon and nutmeg. Try using it in spice breads, muffins, cakes and cookies.

applesauce-spice bread

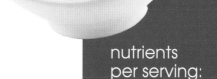

- 1½ cups Gluten-Free All-Purpose Flour Blend (page 5)*
- 1½ cups unsweetened applesauce
- ¾ cup packed light brown sugar
- ½ cup shortening
- 1 teaspoon baking soda
- 1 teaspoon ground cinnamon
- 1 teaspoon vanilla
- ¾ teaspoon xanthan gum
- ½ teaspoon baking powder
- ¼ teaspoon salt
- ¼ teaspoon ground nutmeg
- ½ cup chopped walnuts, toasted**
- ½ cup raisins
- Powdered sugar

*Or use any all-purpose gluten-free flour blend that does not contain xanthan gum.

**To toast walnuts, spread in single layer on baking sheet. Bake in preheated 350°F oven 8 to 10 minutes or until golden brown, stirring frequently.

nutrients per serving:

Calories 337
Calories from Fat 44%
Protein 3g
Carbohydrate 45g
Fiber 2g
Total Fat 17g
Saturated Fat 3g
Cholesterol 0mg
Sodium 239mg

1. Preheat oven to 350°F. Spray 9-inch square baking pan with nonstick cooking spray.

2. Beat flour blend, applesauce, brown sugar, shortening, baking soda, cinnamon, vanilla, xanthan gum, baking powder, salt and nutmeg in large bowl with electric mixer at low speed 30 seconds. Beat at high speed 3 minutes. Stir in walnuts and raisins. Pour into prepared pan.

3. Bake 30 minutes or until toothpick inserted into center comes out clean. Cool completely in pan on wire rack. Sprinkle with powdered sugar before serving.   *Makes 9 servings*

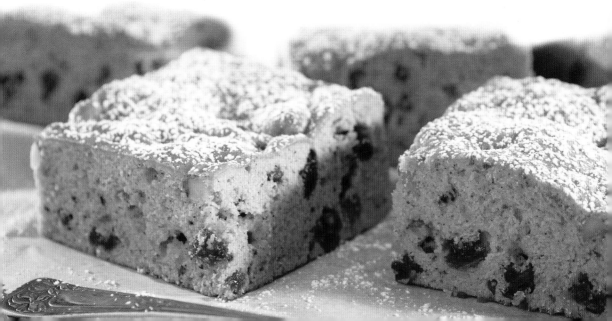

Arborio Rice

Rice is a staple in a gluten-free diet, but Arborio rice goes beyond the basic side dish. This classic Italian ingredient is the star in creamy risotto and can serve as the base of a great meal.

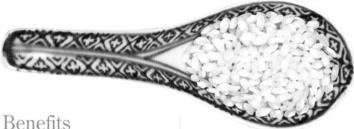

Benefits

Arborio rice is mostly made of carbohydrates, but it does contain a decent amount of protein, more than what is found in the typically eaten long grain white rice. Arborio rice is traditionally used in risotto dishes because its high starch content produces a creamy texture. And it is nearly flavorless, so for someone on a gluten-free diet, it can be used for sweet and savory dishes.

Selection and Storage

Arborio rice is a type of short grain rice traditionally grown in Italy, but it is also grown domestically. It can be purchased in large supermarkets and Italian groceries. Store it in a cool, dry place.

Preparation

Risotto is made by first sautéing this short grain rice in butter or olive oil. A small amount of hot broth is added and the mixture is cooked over low heat with constant stirring until the broth has been absorbed. This process is repeated until all the broth that is called for in the recipe has been added and absorbed. While this may seem a labor intensive, it is one that is worth the effort.

Recipe Suggestions

In Italian cooking, risotto is typically served as a first course or side dish. But in a gluten-free diet, risotto can serve as a great main dish. It has a slightly nutty taste and can be made with a wide variety of ingredients; Parmesan cheese, shellfish, vegetables and herbs are popular additions. Sauces are not needed for risotto because the starches released during cooking give the dish a smooth and rich consistency on its own. You can also get creative and use Arborio rice as a substitute for oatmeal for a rich and creamy breakfast. Just substitute juice for the broth and add any fruits and nuts that complement the flavor of the dish for a sweet and satisfying morning meal. Use Arborio rice in place of long grain rice in rice pudding for an extra creamy, indulgent dessert.

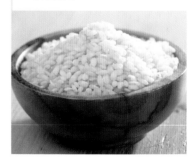

peasant risotto

- 1 tablespoon olive oil
- 3 ounces chopped prosciutto or ham
- 2 cloves garlic, minced
- 1 cup uncooked arborio rice
- 1 can (about 15 ounces) Great Northern beans, rinsed and drained
- ¼ cup chopped green onions
- ½ teaspoon dried sage
- 2 cans (about 14 ounces each) gluten-free reduced-sodium chicken broth, heated
- 1½ cups packed Swiss chard, stemmed and shredded
- ½ cup grated Parmesan cheese

1. Heat oil in large saucepan over medium heat. Add prosciutto and garlic; cook and stir until garlic is browned.

2. Add rice, beans, green onions and sage; cook and stir 2 minutes. Add broth, ½ cup at a time, stirring constantly until all broth is absorbed before adding next ½ cup. Continue until rice is tender and mixture is creamy, about 25 minutes.

3. Stir in Swiss chard and cheese. Remove from heat; cover and let stand 2 minutes or until Swiss chard is wilted. Serve immediately. *Makes 4 servings*

nutrients per serving:

Calories 409
Calories from Fat 19%
Protein 24g
Carbohydrate 60g
Fiber 6g
Total Fat 9g
Saturated Fat 3g
Cholesterol 27mg
Sodium 852mg

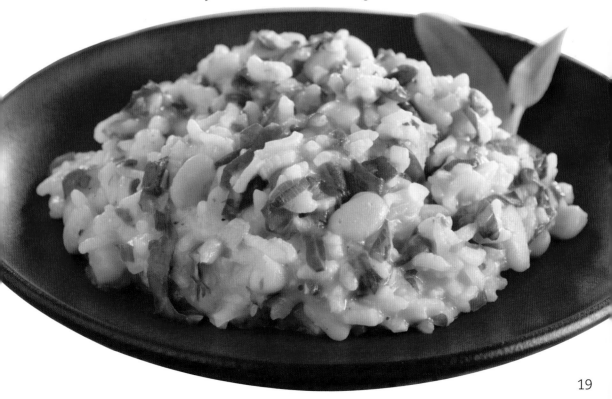

Arrowroot

When it comes to thickening agents, cornstarch and flour are the most commonly used ingredients, however, arrowroot fits the bill, too.

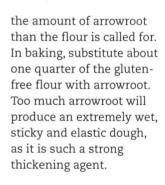

Benefits

Arrowroot is a powder that is ground from a tropical tuber, also called arrowroot. It works just like cornstarch in cooking and baking, acting as a thickener without providing any flavor. Arrowroot can also be used in place of all-purpose flour and has about twice the thickening power, so it works well when used as a substitute in recipes like soups or gravies that may otherwise be gluten-free. What makes it such a great substitute is that it contributes no flavor whatsoever. Arrowroot works in gluten-free baking too, as its thickening characteristic also allows it to act as a binding agent. Moreover, it provides a crisp and light texture that isn't commonly seen in gluten-free baked goods. And for those who do not tolerate gluten-free baked goods well, arrowroot has been known to be easy on the stomach.

Selection and Storage

Arrowroot can be found at natural food stores in the baking aisle or ordered online. Once opened, store tightly covered in the refrigerator.

Preparation

Generally, 2 teaspoons of arrowroot can be used in place of 1 tablespoon of cornstarch. To substitute for the all-purpose flour that is used as a thickener in a recipe, use about one third of the amount of arrowroot than the flour is called for. In baking, substitute about one quarter of the gluten-free flour with arrowroot. Too much arrowroot will produce an extremely wet, sticky and elastic dough, as it is such a strong thickening agent.

Recipe Suggestions

Try using arrowroot in gravies, sauces and soups. It is the recommended thickener for an acidic liquid, but it should not be used for thickening dairy-based recipes because it produces a slimy texture. Use arrowroot when you want to give food a transparent high gloss, such as for a fruit filling in pies or cobblers.

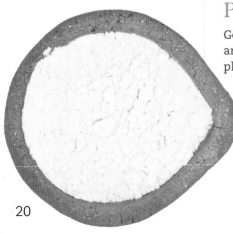

lemony arrowroot cookies

Cookies

- ¼ cup (½ stick) butter
- ⅓ cup granulated sugar
- 1 egg
  Grated peel and juice of 1 lemon
- ½ teaspoon vanilla
- 1¼ cups Gluten-Free All-Purpose Flour Blend (page 5),* plus additional for work surface
- ½ cup arrowroot
- ½ teaspoon baking powder
- ¼ teaspoon salt

Glaze

- ¼ cup powdered sugar
- 1 teaspoon grated lemon peel, plus additional for garnish
- 1 tablespoon lemon juice, plus additional if necessary

*Or use any all-purpose gluten-free flour blend that does not contain xanthan gum.

1. Preheat oven to 350°F. Grease baking sheet.

2. Beat butter and granulated sugar in large bowl with electric mixer at medium speed until creamy. Add egg, grated peel and juice of 1 lemon and vanilla; beat until well blended. Add 1¼ cups flour blend, arrowroot, baking powder and salt; beat at low speed just until combined.

3. Roll dough out onto floured surface to ⅛-inch thickness. Cut out shapes with desired cookie cutters. Place on prepared baking sheet.

4. Bake 8 to 10 minutes. (Cookies will not brown.) Remove to wire rack; cool completely.

5. Combine powdered sugar and 1 teaspoon lemon peel in small bowl; stir in enough lemon juice to make pourable glaze. Drizzle glaze over cookies. Garnish with additional lemon peel.

Makes 12 cookies (1 cookie per serving)

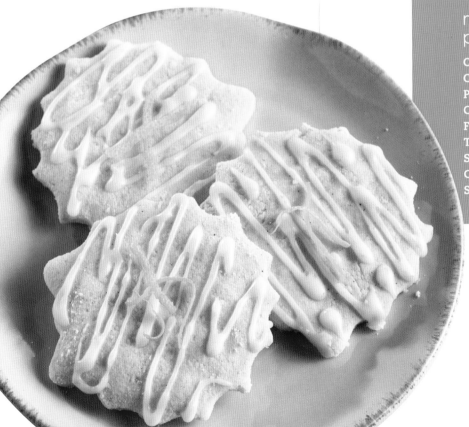

nutrients per serving:

Calories 127
Calories from Fat 38%
Protein 2g
Carbohydrate 18g
Fiber <1g
Total Fat 6g
Saturated Fat 3g
Cholesterol 26mg
Sodium 110mg

Artichokes

This popular and versatile Mediterranean vegetable is a great addition to any diet. With a buttery, delicate flavor, artichokes add a ton of taste and plenty of nutrients to virtually any dish.

Benefits

Artichokes are filled with nutrients that may be deficient in a gluten-free diet, particularly folate. Folate is an important vitamin that is often added to gluten-containing processed foods like cereals, so finding food sources of folate is important for someone on a gluten-free diet. Compared to the artichoke heart, the meaty leaves contain more nutrients.

Selection and Storage

Globe artichokes are commonly available in the produce department. Baby artichokes come from a side thistle of the plant and are available in frozen packages. Artichoke hearts are the most common form of artichokes eaten. The hearts are the meaty base of a whole artichoke and are readily available in cans or marinated in jars. Either frozen baby artichokes or canned artichoke hearts can easily be used in place of fresh in many dishes. Look for fresh artichokes with a soft green color and tightly packed, closed leaves. Store artichokes in a plastic bag in the refrigerator, adding a few drops of water to prevent them from drying out. Although best if used within a few days, they'll keep for a week or two if stored properly.

Preparation

Wash fresh, whole artichokes under cool running water. Pull off outer, lower petals and trim the sharp tips off the outer leaves. Boil artichokes in a saucepan for 20 to 40 minutes or steam them for 25 to 40 minutes or until a center petal pulls out easily and the bottoms are tender when pierced with a fork. They can also be cooked in the microwave. Wrap whole artichokes individually in heavy-duty plastic wrap. Place each wrapped artichoke, bottom side up, in a small shallow bowl or cup. Microwave on HIGH for 12 to 14 minutes, turning and rearranging each artichoke halfway through cooking time.

Recipe Suggestions

Artichokes can be served hot or cold. Try dipping artichoke leaves in melted butter or olive oil and lemon juice. Add artichoke hearts to casseroles or throw them in a salad.

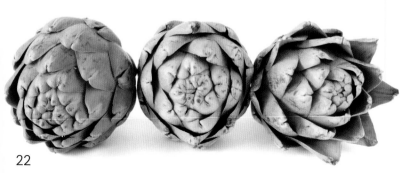

artichokes with lemon-tarragon butter

6 cups water

2¼ teaspoons salt, divided

2 whole artichokes, stems cut off and leaf tips trimmed

¼ cup (½ stick) butter

¼ teaspoon grated lemon peel

2 tablespoons lemon juice

¼ teaspoon dried tarragon

¼ teaspoon salt

1. Bring water and 2 teaspoons salt to a boil in large saucepan over high heat. Add artichokes; return to a boil. Reduce heat to medium-low; cover and simmer 35 to 45 minutes or until leaves detach easily.

2. Turn artichokes upside down to drain well. Cut artichokes in half and remove the fuzzy choke at the bottom that covers the artichoke heart with a spoon.

3. Combine butter, lemon peel, lemon juice, tarragon and remaining ¼ teaspoon salt in small saucepan; heat over low heat until butter is melted. Serve in small bowls for dipping. *Makes 2 servings*

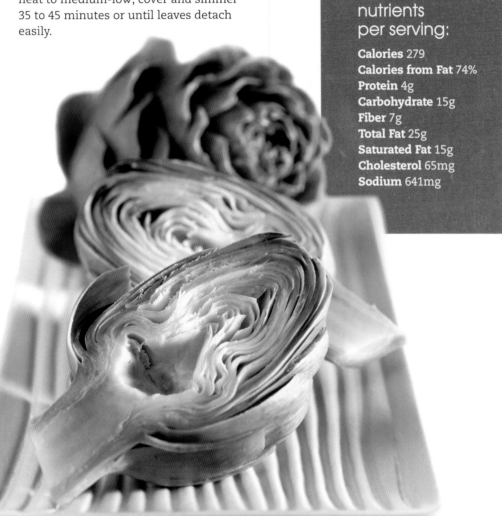

nutrients per serving:

Calories 279
Calories from Fat 74%
Protein 4g
Carbohydrate 15g
Fiber 7g
Total Fat 25g
Saturated Fat 15g
Cholesterol 65mg
Sodium 641mg

Asparagus

Whether you enjoy the typical green, brightly colored purple or plain white variety, this vegetable is always a hit, no matter how it's prepared.

Benefits

Many gluten-free dieters struggle to find foods that work within their limits and also help to maintain their waistline. At less than 4 calories a spear, asparagus is a must for those watching their weight, too. Not only is it low in fat and calories, it is rich in potassium, niacin, and vitamins A and C.

Selection and Storage

Most of the asparagus available in American markets is green. The purple variety is rare and readily available in European markets and farmers' markets. The white variety, sometimes called Belgian asparagus, is even more difficult to find. For the typical green variety, look for it in early spring. Choose asparagus that has a bright green color, stalks that are smooth, firm, straight and round, as well as tips that are compact, closed, pointed and purplish in color. In a bunch, choose stalks of similar size so they'll cook at the same rate. Asparagus will keep for almost a week when wrapped loosely in a plastic bag in the vegetable drawer. To enjoy asparagus year-round, blanch the fresh spears, store them in freezer bags and freeze for up to eight months. Cut or whole spears are also available frozen and canned.

Preparation

Rinse asparagus thoroughly. Snap off the whitish stem ends, and add these to soup stock instead of tossing them out. Boil, steam or microwave the spears, but avoid overcooking. Cooked correctly, the spears should be crisp-tender and bright green. Overcooked spears are mushy and drab olive green. You may have heard of peeling asparagus, which is not necessary, although it does improve the texture of the stems and allows them to cook as quickly as the tender tips.

Recipe Suggestions

Serve asparagus as a hot side dish or in a cold salad. Try adding cut-up spears to your next stir-fry or pasta dish. They work well for breakfast when cooked in egg dishes like frittatas and omelets, too. Or let the flavor of fresh asparagus shine on its own, as it is great grilled or oven-roasted with a light brushing of olive oil and sprinkle of salt and black pepper.

Avocado

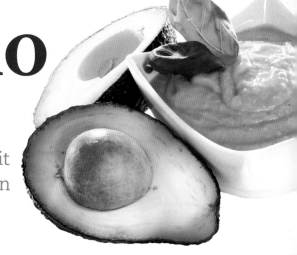

Avocado, native to Mexico, is often mistaken for a vegetable. This rich, smooth-textured fruit is most widely recognized when mashed, seasoned and served as guacamole.

Benefits

Avocado has a rich, buttery flavor that complements many vegetables and meats, especially when added to sandwiches or salads. Puréed, they form the base for soups and sauces. And because of their soft texture, mild taste and pool of vitamins and minerals, they are a fine early food for infants. What also makes them a great first food for infants is what makes them good in a gluten-free diet, too—avocado has been known to be easy on the stomach.

Selection and Storage

Avocados are available year-round. The two most common varieties of

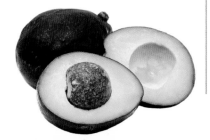

avocados are the pebbly textured, dark-colored Haas and the green Fuerte, with its thin, smooth skin. Ripe avocados yield to gentle pressure and should be unblemished and heavy for their size. Choose firm avocados if you do not plan on using them right away. To speed up ripening, place avocados in a brown bag on the counter. Once ripened, they can be stored in the refrigerator for several days.

Preparation

To prepare an avocado, insert a utility knife into the stem end. Slice in half lengthwise to the pit, turning the avocado while slicing. Remove the knife and twist the halves in opposite directions to pull apart. Press the knife into the pit, twisting gently to pull the pit away from the avocado. Then, peel the skin away or scoop out the flesh with a spoon. Once

avocado is cut and exposed to air, it browns rapidly. Adding the avocado to a dish at the last moment can help minimize this, as can tossing cut avocado with lemon or lime juice. While it will not last long, you can store an avocado half for future use. Sprinkle the surface with lemon or lime juice, wrap tightly in plastic wrap and store in the refrigerator.

Recipe Suggestions

Avocados should be served raw because they have a bitter taste when cooked. To use them in a hot dish, add them just before serving. Try adding sliced avocado to a grilled sandwich or a salad. Combine mashed avocado with chile peppers, cilantro, lime juice, salt and any other desired ingredients, like mango or jicama, to make your own guacamole.

Bananas

Grown in the tropics, bananas are one of the most popular fruits in the United States. Thanks to their handy, easy-open package, they make the perfect take-along gluten-free snack.

Benefits

Eating out or eating on the run isn't easy for people following a gluten-free diet, but you can now find bananas at almost any fast food chain, restaurant, bakery or coffee shop. Even the local drug stores and pharmacies are stocked full of them—so you can always count on finding something to eat when you are pressed for gluten-free options. And they are full of fiber, so they will leave you feeling satisfied until your next meal. Besides being great for their portability, bananas' natural sweet flavor, creamy texture and high moisture content are what make them perfect for use in baked goods, too.

Selection and Storage

There are different types of bananas, but Cavendish, the yellow bananas, are the most common. Look for plump, firm bananas with no bruises or split skins. Brown spots found on bananas indicate ripening. Allow them to ripen at room temperature, refrigerating once they are ripe to stop the process.

Preparation

Sprinkle lemon juice on banana slices to keep them from darkening. Most bananas ripen after picking, and as they do, the starch in them turns to sugar. So the riper they are, the sweeter they are. Overripe bananas are best used in cakes, quick breads and muffins. To mash bananas, use a fork, potato masher or food processor.

To salvage bananas that are too ripe, peel and freeze them so they'll be ready for smoothies or, once thawed, you can also use them for baking.

Recipe Suggestions

Not only do bananas make an easy-to-grab snack or breakfast item, they have many uses when combined with other foods. Smoothies are an excellent snack or meal option for gluten-free dieters. Virtually any combination of fruits, juices and/or yogurt can be used without having to worry about gluten-free ingredients. You can then take any remaining smoothie and pour into a small paper or plastic cup and freeze for your own homemade frozen pop. For a fancier gluten-free treat, sauté sliced bananas in melted butter with some brown sugar and cinnamon. Enjoy sautéed bananas on their own, as a breakfast topper on pancakes or french toast or for dessert over ice cream.

cocoa bottom banana pecan bars

1 cup sugar
½ cup (1 stick) margarine
5 ripe bananas, mashed
1 egg
1 teaspoon vanilla
1½ cups Gluten-Free All-Purpose Flour Blend (page 5)*
1 teaspoon baking powder
1 teaspoon baking soda
½ teaspoon xanthan gum
½ teaspoon salt
½ cup chopped pecans
¼ cup unsweetened cocoa powder

*Or use any all-purpose gluten-free flour blend that does not contain xanthan gum.

1. Preheat oven to 350°F. Grease 13×9-inch baking pan.

2. Beat sugar and margarine in large bowl with electric mixer at medium speed until creamy. Add bananas, egg and vanilla; beat until well blended. Combine flour blend, baking powder, baking soda, xanthan gum and salt in medium bowl. Add to banana mixture; beat until well blended. Stir in pecans.

3. Remove half of batter to another bowl; stir in cocoa. Spread chocolate batter in prepared pan. Top with plain batter; swirl gently with knife.

4. Bake 30 to 35 minutes or until edges are lightly browned. Cool completely in pan on wire rack. Cut into bars.

Makes 2 dozen bars

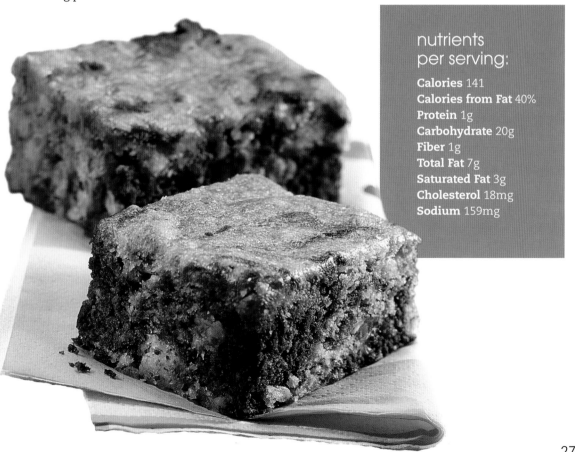

nutrients per serving:

Calories 141
Calories from Fat 40%
Protein 1g
Carbohydrate 20g
Fiber 1g
Total Fat 7g
Saturated Fat 3g
Cholesterol 18mg
Sodium 159mg

Beans

Dried beans are seeds of plants called legumes and come in a variety of shapes, colors and sizes. They enrich almost any meal with a hefty amount of protein and fiber.

Benefits

There are hundreds of varieties of beans available. They are often interchangeable in recipes and easily take on the seasoning of any dish, making them a valuable addition to any diet. They are packed with important nutrients, too. According to research, diets that include beans are associated with lower risks of heart disease and some cancers. This may be due in part to their high amounts of fiber, folate, manganese, magnesium, iron, copper and potassium. Plus, they are packed with protein, making them a great meat alternative for vegetarians or those looking to cut some meat out of their diet.

Selection and Storage

Dried beans are inexpensive, but they require more time to prepare. Dried beans last for a year or more in an airtight container. Store cooked beans for up to one week in the refrigerator or freeze for up to six months. For convenience, you'll find many types of cooked beans available in cans. Be sure to rinse canned beans well to reduce the amount of added sodium by as much as 40 percent.

Preparation

Rinse dried beans under cool running water and pick out any debris or blemished beans. You can either soak the beans overnight or use a quick-soak method. To soak overnight, place beans in a large saucepan or bowl and cover with 3 inches of water. Let stand, covered, for at least 6 hours. Drain, rinse and prepare according to recipe directions. To quick-soak dried beans, place them in a large saucepan and cover with 3 inches of water. Bring to a boil over high heat and boil for 2 minutes. Remove the pan from the heat and let stand 1 to 2 hours before draining, rinsing and proceeding with recipe directions.

Recipe Suggestions

Beans make an excellent meat alternative or side dish. Try adding them to salads, soups or stews. One popular preparation is puréeing them for a vegetable dip or spread. Hummus may be the best-known dip, which is traditionally made with puréed chickpeas (also known as garbanzo beans). However, different types of beans work just as well.

black bean dip

- **1 can (about 15 ounces) refried black beans**
- **½ cup chunky salsa**
- **½ cup cream cheese**
- **½ cup (2 ounces) shredded Monterey Jack cheese**
- **½ teaspoon ground cumin**
- **½ cup chopped fresh cilantro or green onions**
  Bell pepper strips or corn tortilla chips (optional)

Slow Cooker Directions

1. Combine beans, salsa, cream cheese, Monterey Jack cheese and cumin in slow cooker. Cover; cook on HIGH 1½ to 2 hours or until heated through, stirring once after 1 hour.

2. Stir in cilantro. Serve with bell pepper strips or tortilla chips, if desired.   *Makes 8 servings*

nutrients per serving:

Calories 139
Calories from Fat 54%
Protein 6g
Carbohydrate 10g
Fiber 3g
Total Fat 9g
Saturated Fat 4g
Cholesterol 23mg
Sodium 340mg

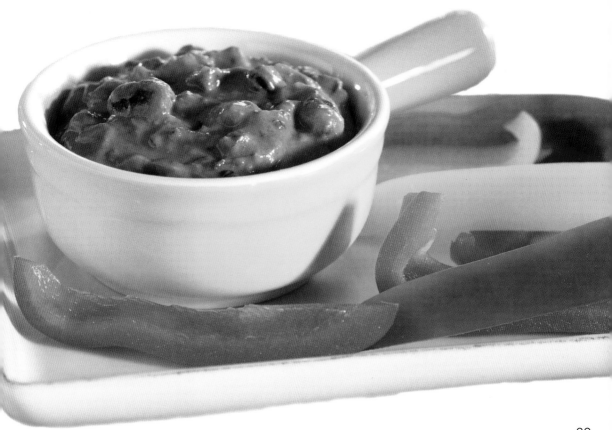

Beef

Benefits

Beef is filled with high-quality protein and essential vitamins and minerals. If you are concerned about calorie and fat counts, purchase cuts with "loin" or "round" in the name. Beef tenderloin contains only 8 grams of fat and 170 calories per 3-ounce serving, less than a skinless chicken thigh. Try and use grass-fed beef, as it has been found to be more nutritious than corn-fed beef, containing higher amounts of vitamin E and omega-3 fatty acids while also being lower in calories and saturated fat.

Selection and Storage

Choose beef with a bright cherry-red or purplish color without any gray or brown blotches. Use refrigerated beef within four days after purchase or freeze

It's no wonder beef is so popular in American diets. Whether enjoying a juicy fillet or a mouthwatering burger, this food is loved in so many ways.

soon after purchase if you do not plan on using it right away. Grass-fed beef is harder to find than corn-fed beef, but it is becoming more available as increasing emphasis is placed on its greater health benefits. Look for it in large natural food stores with a good meat selection, at butcher shops or at large farmers' markets.

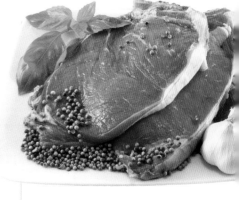

Preparation

To keep beef lean, trim all fat from the exterior. Tender beef cuts, like tenderloin, are best prepared with a dry-heat cooking method, such as roasting, grilling or broiling. When using a marinade, tender cuts of beef will need to marinate for 15 minutes to 2 hours to impart flavor. A seasoning rub is another great way to add flavor to the surface of beef. Just be sure any store-bought prepared marinades,

rubs or seasonings are gluten-free. Cook beef tenderloin to an internal temperature of at least 145°F for medium rare.

Recipe Suggestions

Try grilling, broiling, roasting or braising cuts of beef. Cut beef into chunks and add it to a stir-fry or use in a hearty stew with your favorite vegetables and seasonings. Ground beef is a great versatile food, too. It can be used in countless ways, including for meatballs, burgers, meat loaves, tacos, chilis and casseroles.

beef stew stroganoff

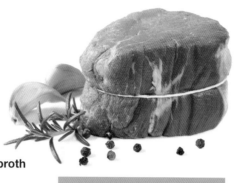

- 2 tablespoons olive oil
- 1½ pounds lean boneless beef (bottom round), cut into 1-inch cubes
- 1 teaspoon caraway seeds
- ½ teaspoon salt
- ½ teaspoon black pepper
- ½ teaspoon dried thyme
- 2 cans (about 14 ounces each) gluten-free beef broth
- 1 cup sliced mushrooms
- ½ cup thinly sliced carrots
- ½ cup chopped red bell pepper
- 6 ounces baby red potatoes, unpeeled, quartered (about 6 small)
- ¼ cup sour cream

1. Heat oil in large saucepan over medium-high heat. Add beef; cook and stir until meat juices evaporate and begin to caramelize. Add caraway seeds, salt, black pepper and thyme. Pour in broth, stirring to scrape up browned bits. Bring to a boil.

2. Add mushrooms, carrots and bell pepper. Reduce heat; cover and simmer 1 hour.

3. Increase heat; add potatoes. Bring to a boil. Reduce heat; cover and simmer 20 minutes.

4. Stir in sour cream; cook 2 minutes or until heated through.   *Makes 6 servings*

nutrients per serving:

Calories 271
Calories from Fat 41%
Protein 29g
Carbohydrate 8g
Fiber 1g
Total Fat 12g
Saturated Fat 4g
Cholesterol 72mg
Sodium 1279mg

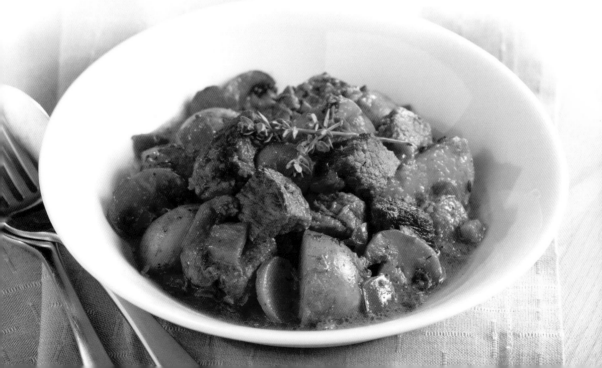

Beets

The bright red color of beets is not the only thing that makes them stand out—they are delicious and highly nutritious no matter how you enjoy them.

Benefits

Beets, which have a sweet, earthy flavor, can be cooked and eaten in many ways: warm or cold, alone or combined with other ingredients. Additionally, beets are particularly rich in folate, fiber and potassium, important nutrients typically lacking in a gluten-free diet. The attached beet greens are edible and extremely healthful, as well.

Selection and Storage

Choose smaller, firm beets of uniform size. The freshest beets are those topped with bright, crisp greens. The skins should be deep red, smooth and unblemished. Once you get beets home, remove the greens and store them separately in a plastic bag. Leave 2 inches of stems on beets so they don't bleed when cooked. Store beets in the refrigerator for up to two weeks. You can also purchase prepared cooked beets at specialty grocery stores in sealed packages in the refrigerated section near the regular produce. Or, if you plan on using them right away, just visit almost any salad bar to purchase sliced fresh beets. Canned whole, sliced and diced beets are also readily available at any major supermarket.

Preparation

Wash fresh beets gently, as broken skin will allow color and nutrients to escape—and don't peel them before cooking for the same reason. Microwaving retains the most nutrients. You can cook them on the stove, too: Cover with water, bring to a boil and simmer for 25 to 30 minutes. Roasting beets will bring out their sweet flavor. Roast them in a 425°F oven for about 45 minutes or until tender when pierced with a fork. When slicing cooled cooked beets, use a glass plate because the beet juice will stain wood and plastic cutting boards. Beet greens can be cooked and served like spinach or Swiss chard.

Recipe Suggestions

Beets can be cooked and served as a side dish, or pickled or roasted for a salad. They are the main ingredient in borscht, a popular European soup. Their sweet flavor complements tangy ingredients. Try warm cooked beets with a mustard sauce or toss chilled sliced beets in your favorite salad with some feta or goat cheese.

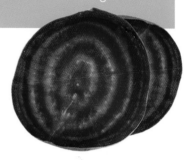

beets in spicy mustard sauce

3 pounds beets, trimmed
¼ cup reduced-fat sour cream
2 tablespoons spicy brown mustard
2 teaspoons lemon juice
2 cloves garlic, minced
¼ teaspoon black pepper
⅛ teaspoon dried thyme

1. Place beets in large saucepan; add enough water to cover by
1 inch. Bring to a boil over medium-high heat. Reduce heat to
medium-low; cover and simmer 25 minutes or until tender. Drain
well. Peel beets; cut into ¼-inch-thick slices.

2. Combine sour cream, mustard, lemon juice, garlic, pepper and
thyme in small saucepan; cook and stir over medium heat until
heated through. Spoon sauce over beets; toss gently to coat.

Makes 4 servings

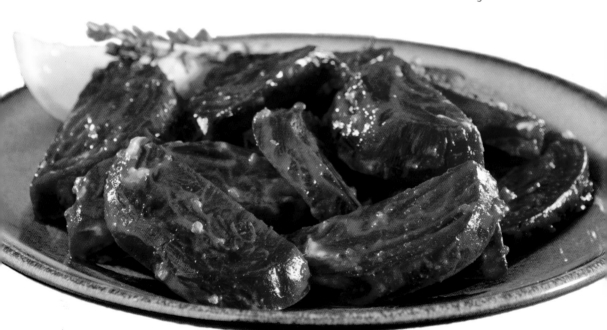

Bell Peppers

Hundreds of pepper varieties exist in a multitude of shapes, sizes and colors, yet the sweet bell pepper—known for its bell-like shape—is the most common type eaten today.

Benefits

Bell peppers, or sweet peppers, come in a spectrum of hues from vibrant green to deep red, depending on variety and stage of ripeness. They're perfect for adding color, flavor and crunch to a variety of dishes. They are also bursting with nutrients, including vitamins A and C, antioxidants that help prevent cell damage, inflammation, cancer and age-related diseases, as well as help support immune functions. They additionally provide a decent dose of fiber.

Selection and Storage

Green peppers are simply red, orange or yellow peppers that have yet to ripen. As they ripen, they get sweeter and turn various shades until they reach their mature color.

Once ripe, they are more perishable, so they carry a premium price. Regardless of age, bell peppers should have a glossy sheen and no shriveling, cracks or soft spots. Select those that are heavy for their size. Store bell peppers in a plastic bag in your refrigerator's crisper drawer. Green bell peppers stay firm for a week; other colors go soft in three or four days.

Preparation

Bell peppers should be washed under cold running water before using. To slice or chop bell peppers, stand one on its end on a cutting board. Cut lengthwise slices from the sides, avoiding the stem

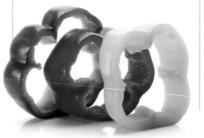

and center. Discard the stem and seeds and scrape out any remaining seeds. You may want to rinse the inside of the bell pepper slices, as well.

Recipe Suggestions

Bell peppers are often eaten raw but can be cooked and added to a host of dishes. Add bell peppers at the end of cooking time because they develop a stronger flavor when cooked; when overcooked, their flavor becomes bitter. Use bell pepper slices to add crunch and color to a salad, as a dipper with guacamole or hummus, or snack on them alone. Try adding bell peppers to stir-fries and casseroles, but be sure to add them at the end to retain the best flavor and texture. Try using hollowed out whole bell peppers to serve tuna, egg, turkey or chicken salad.

Berries

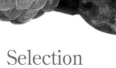

No matter what type of berry you like, you can't go wrong with these sweet-tasting fruits—they are filled with juicy flavor and nutrients.

Benefits

One of the most difficult nutrients for those on a gluten-free diet to get is fiber. Fiber is mostly found in wheat-containing products, but is abundant in plenty of vegetables and fruits and especially high in berries. The seeds of blackberries, strawberries and raspberries are packed with fiber, as are the skins of blueberries. Raspberries contain the most amount of fiber out of all the berries, at an astounding 8 grams per ½ cup serving. Fiber is an important nutrient for everyone, as a diet high in fiber has been found to aid in weight loss and disease prevention, including heart disease and some cancers. But fiber is especially important for those with celiac disease because it helps to strengthen and soothe the digestive tract. For adults and adolescents, the recommended daily amount is 25 to 38 grams per day.

Selection and Storage

Look for blackberries that are glossy, plump, deep colored, firm and well rounded. Choose blueberries that are firm, uniform in size and indigo blue with a silvery frost. Purchase brightly colored raspberries with no hulls attached. Look for plump strawberries that are ruby red and evenly colored with green, leafy tops. All berries should be stored in the refrigerator and used within a day or two of purchasing. Frozen berries, on their own or combined, are readily available at the supermarket.

Preparation

Do not wash berries until you are ready to use them because they are fragile and spoil quickly. Wash berries gently under cool running water and drain well. Sort through berries to remove stems and ones that are soft. Do not overhandle them, or their cells will break open and they will lose their juice and nutrients.

Recipe Suggestions

Adding berries and their important nutrients to your daily diet is easy. Add blueberries or raspberries to your morning bowl of cereal or toss any variety of berry into a cup of yogurt. Top a salad with some sliced strawberries. You can always snack on berries alone, too. Frozen berries work well when combined with yogurt and blended into a smoothie for breakfast or a sweet, satisfying snack. Thawed frozen berries and their juices make a delicious topping for ice cream or sorbet.

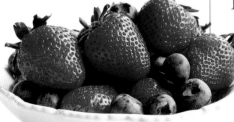

Brown Rice Flour

Brown rice flour is one of the most commonly used gluten-free flours because it's an easy substitute for all-purpose flour when used in small quantities.

Benefits

Rice flour is so popular for gluten-free dieters because it easily replaces all-purpose flour in some recipes. If a small amount of flour is called for to bind ingredients together, rice flour works just as well and can be easily substituted in a one-to-one ratio. Brown rice flour, like the brown rice it is made from, has a slightly better nutritional profile than white rice flour because it is a whole grain, so it offers a fair amount of fiber and protein. Brown and white rice flours can be used interchangeably, but brown rice flour has a deeper, slightly nutty and sweet flavor.

Selection and Storage

Brown rice flour can be found in the gluten-free section of natural food stores. It is available in fine and medium grinds, yet many people prefer the fine grind because the medium one can have a gritty texture. Once the package is opened, it should be stored in an airtight container and refrigerated.

Preparation

Because it is a whole grain, brown rice flour is denser than all-purpose flour and can therefore typically be used as a substitute for recipes calling for very small amounts, like a tablespoon or two. The dense texture does allow it to work as a great thickening agent for soups, roux and gravies. It is also one of the base ingredients in many gluten-free flour blends, including both of the blends in this book, because it contributes a wonderful texture without imparting much flavor.

Recipe Suggestions

Brown rice flour works perfectly in recipes that call for using all-purpose flour as a minor ingredient in a breading or coating, such as for chicken or fish. For a great gluten-free coating, combine gluten-free bread crumbs or cornmeal and any desired seasonings with a few tablespoons of brown rice flour. The dense texture will provide a crispy bite to the food you're cooking. You can also try combining ground nuts, like pecans, with a few tablespoons of brown rice flour for another crunchy coating.

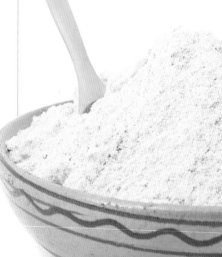

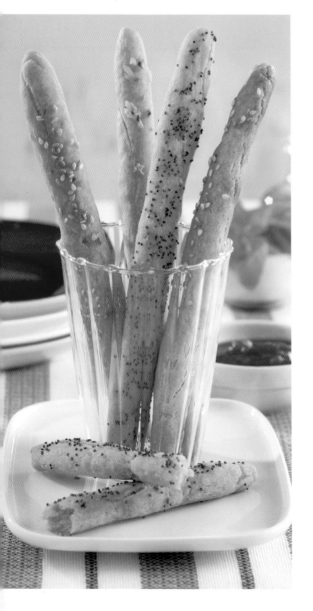

gf breadsticks

3½ cups Gluten-Free Flour Blend for Breads
   (page 5)
  1 package (¼ ounce) active dry yeast
  3 teaspoons salt, divided
1½ teaspoons xanthan gum
  1 teaspoon unflavored gelatin
1⅓ cups warm water
  2 tablespoons olive oil
  1 tablespoon honey

Garlic Topping
  2 tablespoons olive oil
  2 to 4 cloves garlic, minced

1. Place flour blend, yeast, 2 teaspoons salt, xanthan gum and gelatin in food processor; process until mixed. With processor running, add water, 2 tablespoons oil and honey. Process 30 seconds or until thoroughly combined. (Dough will be sticky.) Transfer to large greased bowl.

2. Shape dough into rough ball with damp hands. Cover; let rise in warm place 45 minutes. Punch down dough; let rest 15 minutes.

3. Preheat oven to 450°F. Line baking sheets with parchment paper. Place 1½-inch portions of dough on clean surface; roll into 8-inch-long breadsticks. Transfer to prepared baking sheets.

4. Bake 10 minutes. Meanwhile, combine 2 tablespoons oil and garlic in small bowl. Remove breadsticks from oven; brush garlic topping onto breadsticks.

5. Bake 10 minutes or until browned. Remove to wire racks to cool slightly. Serve warm.

Makes 15 to 20 breadsticks
(1 breadstick per serving)

Variation: For a sesame seed or poppy seed topping, brush breadsticks lightly with water and sprinkle evenly with seeds before baking.

Tip: Be sure to rotate pans once during baking so that the breadsticks brown evenly.

Buckwheat

Despite its name, buckwheat is not a type of wheat, nor is it a grain; it's the seed from an herb. It has a nutty flavor and serves many purposes in a gluten-free diet.

Benefits

Buckwheat is enjoyed in many ways, including ground into flour, crushed into groats or grits, or roasted as kasha. Plus, it is a nutrition powerhouse. Buckwheat is high in protein and a good source of fiber, a nutrient often missing from a gluten-free diet. A phytochemical in buckwheat called rutin is a known cancer fighter and helps to reduce cholesterol levels and strengthen blood vessels.

Selection and Storage

When buckwheat is hulled and crushed, it's called groats. You can buy groats cracked into coarse, medium or fine grinds. Roasted groats, or kasha, can be found in all grinds in the Kosher section of the supermarket. Very finely cracked unroasted groats, or buckwheat grits, are sold as hot cereal. Keep buckwheat in a well-sealed container in the refrigerator or freezer. At room temperature, it is susceptible to turning rancid.

Preparation

If you purchase buckwheat in its natural form, be sure to rinse it thoroughly and remove any dirt or debris. Bring 1 cup of buckwheat and 2 cups of liquid, like water or broth, to a boil; reduce the heat to low and cover and simmer for about 30 minutes or until all of the liquid is absorbed. Cook groats or kasha like rice, following package instructions for the amount of water. Typically, 1 cup of kasha will require 3 to 4 cups of cooking liquid, depending on the desired consistency of the dish you are making. Bring the kasha and liquid to a boil; reduce the heat and cook and stir for 8 to 10 minutes or until all the liquid is absorbed.

Recipe Suggestions

You can substitute buckwheat groats or kasha in most recipes calling for rice or other whole grains. Kasha is used in traditional Jewish dishes and can be found at almost any Jewish deli in chicken soup or as a filling for a knish (a potato dumpling). The fine grinds make a deliciously creamy hot cereal with a wonderful nutty flavor. For a welcome change, try using finely ground kasha in place of oats in almost any recipe.

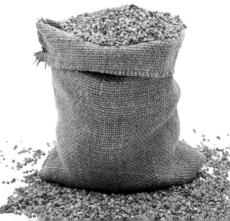

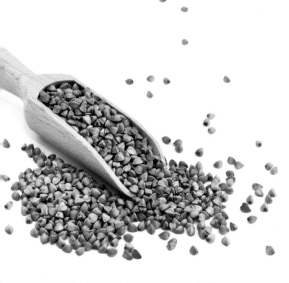

buckwheat breakfast bowl

3 to 4 cups reduced-fat (2%) milk*
2 tablespoons packed brown sugar
½ teaspoon vanilla
½ teaspoon ground cinnamon, divided
1 cup kasha
2 teaspoons butter
2 apples, cut into ½-inch chunks
2 tablespoons maple syrup
¼ cup chopped walnuts

*For a creamier consistency, use more milk.

1. Combine milk, brown sugar, vanilla and ¼ teaspoon cinnamon in large saucepan. Bring to a boil over medium heat. Stir in kasha; reduce heat to low. Cook and stir 8 to 10 minutes or until kasha is tender and liquid is absorbed.

2. Meanwhile, melt butter in large nonstick skillet over medium heat. Stir in remaining ¼ teaspoon cinnamon. Add apples; cook and stir 4 to 5 minutes or until tender. Stir in maple syrup and walnuts; heat through.

3. Spoon kasha into six bowls. Top with apple mixture. Serve immediately.   *Makes 6 servings*

nutrients per serving:

Calories 226
Calories from Fat 32%
Protein 6g
Carbohydrate 34g
Fiber 3g
Total Fat 8g
Saturated Fat 3g
Cholesterol 13mg
Sodium 119mg

kasha vegetable soup

2 tablespoons olive oil
1 package (8 ounces) sliced mushrooms
1 medium onion, chopped
1 cup chopped celery
1 cup chopped carrots
2 cloves garlic, minced
8 cups gluten-free vegetable broth
1 teaspoon salt
1 teaspoon black pepper
½ teaspoon dried thyme
1 bay leaf
½ cup kasha

nutrients per serving:

Calories 93
Calories from Fat 40%
Protein 4g
Carbohydrate 10g
Fiber 2g
Total Fat 4g
Saturated Fat <1g
Cholesterol 0mg
Sodium 886mg

1. Heat oil in large saucepan or Dutch oven over medium heat. Add mushrooms, onion, celery, carrots and garlic; cook and stir 7 to 10 minutes or until vegetables are tender.

2. Add broth, salt, pepper, thyme and bay leaf. Bring to a boil. Reduce heat to low; cover and simmer 30 minutes.

3. Stir in kasha; cook 10 minutes or until kasha is tender. Remove and discard bay leaf before serving.   *Makes 8 servings*

Buckwheat Flour

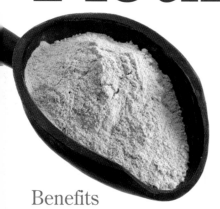

Buckwheat flour is best known for the robust, slightly nutty pancakes it produces. For people on gluten-free diets, buckwheat flour offers a delicious way to enjoy this favorite morning comfort food.

Benefits

Ground from whole grain buckwheat, this flour is especially high in protein and fiber. It has more protein than most grains, and the protein is more nutritionally complete. Buckwheat flour is enjoyed for its nutritional heft as well as its hearty taste. It makes a satisfying substitution for wheat flour in pancakes and crêpes. Buckwheat flour is also made into Japanese soba noodles, providing a welcome alternative to the more neutral-tasting gluten-free pastas that are available.

Selection and Storage

Buckwheat flour is most often found among specialty flours in large supermarkets or natural food stores, usually near other gluten-free foods. Make sure you select packages of only buckwheat flour, as some brands also sell buckwheat-wheat flour blends and buckwheat pancake mixes in similar looking packages. Store it in the refrigerator or freezer, where it will stay fresh for several months.

Preparation

When starting to cook with buckwheat flour, begin with simple pancakes or crêpes. You may use all buckwheat flour or else half buckwheat flour and half other gluten-free flour, such as quinoa flour or even a blend for quick breads. For something a little more adventurous, try blini, which are Russian pancakes that are similar to crêpes but leavened with yeast. They are traditionally served with sour cream and caviar or smoked salmon. If you're looking to branch out, be aware that buckwheat is not recommended for use in most breads and baked goods. Because it contains no gluten, it lacks the necessary structure when there is no wheat flour present.

Recipe Suggestions

Try adding your favorite berries to pancake batter and top finished pancakes with butter and maple syrup for a breakfast treat. You may notice that buckwheat pancakes are darker in color than regular, and even take on a blue tint. The possibilities for crêpes are endless, going either sweet or savory and suitable for breakfast, brunch, lunch and even dinner. For sweet, try filling crêpes with chocolate-hazelnut spread and fresh strawberries. For savory, fill them with goat cheese and some chopped fresh herbs.

buckwheat pancakes

- 1 cup buckwheat flour
- 2 tablespoons cornstarch
- 2 teaspoons baking powder
- ¼ teaspoon salt
- ¼ teaspoon ground cinnamon
- 1 cup whole milk
- 1 egg
- 2 tablespoons butter, melted
- 2 tablespoons maple syrup
- ½ teaspoon vanilla
  - **Additional butter for cooking**
  - **Additional maple syrup (optional)**

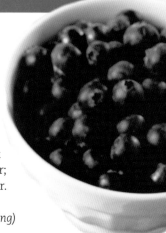

nutrients per serving:

Calories 251	**Total Fat** 10g
Calories from Fat 35%	**Saturated Fat** 5g
Protein 7g	**Cholesterol** 68mg
Carbohydrate 35g	**Sodium** 489mg
Fiber 3g	

1. Whisk buckwheat flour, cornstarch, baking powder, salt and cinnamon in medium bowl. Combine milk, egg, 2 tablespoons butter, 2 tablespoons maple syrup and vanilla in small bowl. Whisk into dry ingredients just until combined. Let stand 5 minutes. (Batter will be thick and elastic.)

2. Heat additional butter in griddle or large nonstick skillet over medium heat. Pour ¼ cupfuls batter 2 inches apart onto griddle. Cook 2 minutes or until lightly browned and edges begin to bubble. Turn over; cook 2 minutes or until lightly browned. Repeat with remaining batter. Serve with additional maple syrup, if desired.

Makes 12 pancakes (3 pancakes per serving)

Variation: Add ½ cup blueberries to the batter.

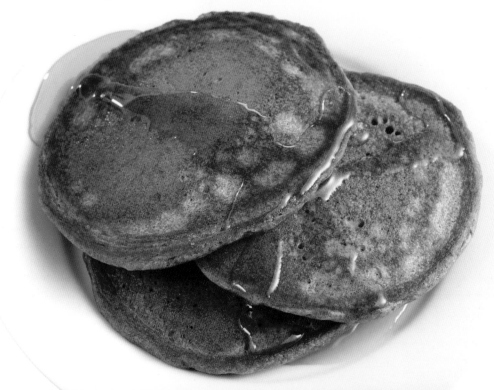

Butternut Squash

Sweet and buttery tasting, this satisfying and fiber-rich winter squash is an excellent addition to any meal and is delicious with many sweet and savory ingredients.

Benefits

Butternut squash has been gaining popularity because of its wonderful flavor, versatile uses and hefty nutrient profile. It is simply bursting with essential vitamins and minerals. It is filled with fiber, and its deep orange color indicates it is rich in beta-carotene, a form of vitamin A that plays an important role in eye and skin health.

Selection and Storage

Butternut squash is available year-round, but its peak season is from early fall through winter. It has a bulbous end and smooth outer shell that ranges from yellow to camel colored. Choose a squash that is firm and free of bruises, punctures or cuts. Butternut squash can be stored in a cool, dark place for many weeks. Its tough shell allows for longer storage so you can enjoy it well into the winter and early spring months.

Preparation

The simplest way to prepare butternut squash is to cut it in half and bake or microwave it. Because the skin is so tough, use caution and a sharp knife to cut the squash. To help soften it for easier cutting, pierce the skin with a fork and microwave on HIGH for 3 to 5 minutes. Let the squash cool for a few minutes before cutting. Then, cut it lengthwise, scoop out the seeds and proceed with cooking or peeling.

Recipe Suggestions

Add cubed squash to soups or stews. Or try it mashed as an alternative to sweet potatoes. Roasting butternut squash really brings out the flavor and makes a delicious side dish. Slice the squash in half lengthwise, scoop out the seeds and place on a baking sheet, skin side down. Roast for about 45 minutes in a 400°F oven, basting the flesh with a little melted butter or olive oil. Try it with almost any combination of savory spices, like curry powder and thyme. For a sweeter side dish, sprinkle it with some brown sugar and cinnamon.

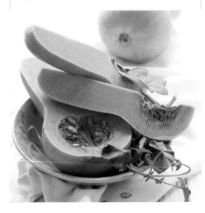

butternut bisque

1 teaspoon margarine or butter
1 large onion, coarsely chopped
1 medium butternut squash (about
 1½ pounds), cut into ½-inch
 pieces
2 cans (about 14 ounces each)
 gluten-free reduced-sodium
 chicken broth, divided
½ teaspoon ground nutmeg
⅛ teaspoon white pepper
 Plain nonfat yogurt and chopped
 chives (optional)

1. Melt margarine in large saucepan over medium heat. Add onion; cook and stir 3 minutes. Add squash and 1 can broth; bring to a boil over high heat. Reduce heat to low; cover and simmer 20 minutes or until squash is very tender.

2. Purée soup in batches in blender, returning blended soup to saucepan after each batch.* (Or use hand-held immersion blender.) Add remaining can of broth, nutmeg and pepper. Simmer, uncovered, 5 minutes, stirring occasionally.

3. Ladle soup into serving bowls. Serve with yogurt and chives, if desired.
Makes 6 (¾-cup) servings

Use caution when processing hot liquids in blender. Vent lid of blender and cover with clean kitchen towel.

Variation: Add ½ cup whipping cream or half-and-half with the second can of broth.

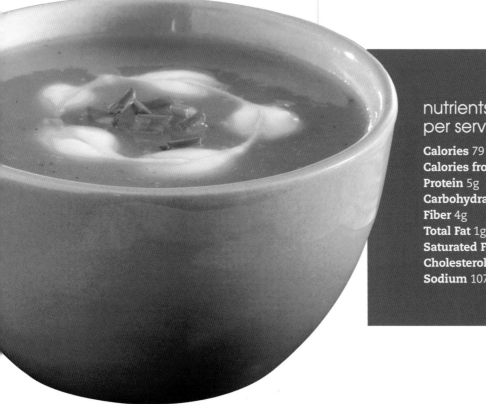

nutrients per serving:

Calories 79
Calories from Fat 9%
Protein 5g
Carbohydrate 14g
Fiber 4g
Total Fat 1g
Saturated Fat <1g
Cholesterol 0mg
Sodium 107mg

Carrots

There aren't many foods that are superior to carrots. With their vibrant color, versatility, great taste and beneficial nutrients, carrots are an easy food to enjoy.

Benefits

Besides being delicious to eat, carrots are good for your body, too. While most vegetables lose vitamins and other healthy nutrients during cooking, carrots are an exception. Cooking carrots actually causes more nutrients to be released for the body to use, like beta-carotene. Beta-carotene is an antioxidant that may help prevent cancer and other diseases. In fact, a mere ½ cup serving of carrots packs a huge amount of this antioxidant form of vitamin A.

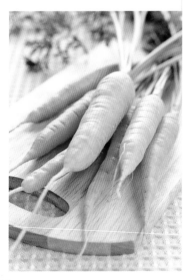

Selection and Storage

Look for firm carrots with bright orange color and smooth skins. Avoid those that are limp or black near the tops. Choose medium-size carrots that taper at the ends; thicker ones may be tough. Baby-cut carrots are sweet and provide all the nutrients plus added convenience. Store carrots in the refrigerator up to two weeks.

Preparation

You can find carrots in a variety of shapes and sizes, precut, shredded or sliced, in packages in the refrigerated part of the produce section. If you choose to buy whole carrots, thoroughly wash and scrub them to remove soil contaminants. To remove pesticide residues, peel the outer layer and cut off the part near the fat end. You can shred fresh carrots by hand using the large holes of a grater or with a food processor fitted with a shredding disc. To cook carrots, steam or boil them in a small amount of liquid until crisp-tender.

Recipe Suggestions

Carrots have a light sweet flavor and crisp bite that complement almost any food they are combined with. Mix some shredded carrots into coleslaws, tuna or chicken salads or any lettuce-based salad. Carrot sticks and baby-cut carrots are a great raw snack and can be eaten on their own or with virtually every type of dip, from bean dips to creamy and cheesy dips. The true sweet flavor of carrots shines through when cooked. Use cooked carrots to thicken soups, stews or sauces, or add them to casseroles or side dishes to provide a sweet flavor and added crunch. Shredded carrots work well in baking—including for muffins, cakes and quick breads—due to their high moisture and sugar contents.

Celery

While celery sticks make for a great gluten-free snack—alone or with dips—this crunchy nutrient-packed vegetable has even better uses in cooking.

Benefits

The high water and fiber contents are what give celery its crisp bite, making it filling and satisfying to munch on, no matter if it is raw or cooked. Celery is a decent source of potassium and also contains good amounts of vitamin C and folate. Celery leaves are the most nutritious part of the plant, containing more nutrients than the stalks.

Selection and Storage

Choose tightly formed bunches of celery with bright green leaves. Store celery in a plastic bag in the refrigerator for up to two weeks, leaving the ribs attached to the stalk until ready to use. Prepackaged cut-up celery is available in the refrigerated part of the produce section.

Preparation

Separate celery stalks and rinse them well to remove dirt from the inner stalks. Remove the leaves and save them for use in soups or stews. If you are planning on eating celery raw, you can use a peeler to remove the outer threads or simply pull any tough pieces down the length of the rib.

Recipe Suggestions

Celery sticks are, of course, great for munching on their own or for using with dips. In fact, if you find dining out to be challenging—like most gluten-free dieters do—many restaurants will now provide celery sticks upon request to use in place of bread for appetizers. Raw finely chopped celery is a great, nearly flavorless, way to add a crisp bite to egg, tuna and chicken salads. And chopped celery is a cooking staple; it is often sautéed in a little olive oil or butter with garlic and other vegetables such as carrots and onions as a base for many dishes, including soup stocks, stews and casseroles. Celery maintains its crisp-tender texture when cooked, so it gives a crunch to any dish it is cooked in.

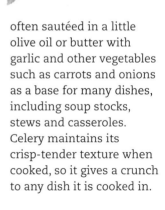

Cellophane Noodles

Cellophane noodles—also called bean thread noodles or glass noodles—are made from powdered mung beans. When cooked, they become transparent and appear to be made of cellophane.

Benefits

Cellophane noodles are clear, thin noodles that are made from mung bean starch and are therefore gluten-free. They are commonly used in Asian cooking but are rather flavorless with a pleasant texture, so they can be used in pasta dishes with any combinations of ingredients and sauces. They are great cold and can be used for pasta salads, too.

Selection and Storage

Cellophane noodles can be found in the Asian section of the supermarket and at Asian markets. They are sold in packages of tangled bunches.

Preparation

Place cellophane noodles in a large bowl, cover with hot water and soak for 15 to 20 minutes or until soft and pliable. Drain the noodles and cut into desired lengths. While cellophane noodles are typically soaked, they can also be fried. To fry them, cut each bundle of noodles in half. Gently pull each half apart into small bunches. Fill a wok or large skillet with vegetable oil and heat the oil over medium-high heat to 375°F on a deep-fry thermometer. Using a slotted spoon or tongs, lower a few small bunches of noodles into the hot oil. Cook 3 to 5 seconds or until noodles rise to the top. Remove immediately and drain on paper towels. Repeat with remaining noodles.

Recipe Suggestions

Make your favorite stir-fry with cellophane noodles by sautéing vegetables with a little bit of peanut or vegetable oil in a wok or large skillet. Add tofu, shrimp or chicken, if you like. Once everything is cooked, add softened cellophane noodles to the wok and stir-fry 1 minute or until heated through. Add uncooked cellophane noodles to soups and let them soften and absorb the flavors of the broth. For a cold salad, toss softened cellophane noodles with a dressing and any other ingredients in a large bowl and cover and refrigerate until ready to serve. Use whatever vegetables, meat or seafood, herbs and nuts you like. A great Asian dressing uses 3 tablespoons rice vinegar, 3 tablespoons soy sauce, 2 tablespoons peanut oil, some freshly grated ginger, chopped cilantro and a sprinkle of lime juice.

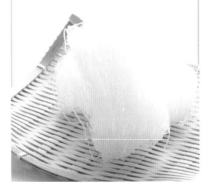

cellophane noodles with minced pork

- 1 package (about 4 ounces) cellophane noodles
- 32 dried shiitake mushrooms
- 2 tablespoons minced fresh ginger
- 2 tablespoons gluten-free black bean sauce
- 1½ cups gluten-free chicken broth
- 1 tablespoon dry sherry
- 1 tablespoon gluten-free soy sauce
- 2 tablespoons vegetable oil
- 6 ounces lean ground pork
- 3 green onions, sliced
- 1 jalapeño or other hot pepper,* finely chopped
- Cilantro sprigs and hot red peppers (optional)

Jalapeño peppers can sting and irritate the skin, so wear rubber gloves when handling peppers and do not touch your eyes.

1. Place cellophane noodles and dried mushrooms in separate bowls; cover each with hot water. Let stand 30 minutes; drain.

2. Cut cellophane noodles into 4-inch pieces. Squeeze out excess water from mushrooms. Cut off and discard mushroom stems; cut caps into thin slices.

3. Combine ginger and black bean sauce in small bowl. Combine broth, sherry and soy sauce in medium bowl.

4. Heat oil in wok or large skillet over high heat. Add pork; stir-fry 2 minutes or until no longer pink. Add green onions, jalapeño and black bean sauce mixture; stir-fry 1 minute.

5. Add broth mixture, cellophane noodles and mushrooms. Simmer, uncovered, about 5 minutes or until most of liquid is absorbed. Garnish with cilantro and red peppers.   *Makes 4 servings*

nutrients per serving:

Calories 372	Total Fat 15g
Calories from Fat 34%	Saturated Fat 4g
Protein 13g	Cholesterol 29mg
Carbohydrate 50g	Sodium 791mg
Fiber 4g	

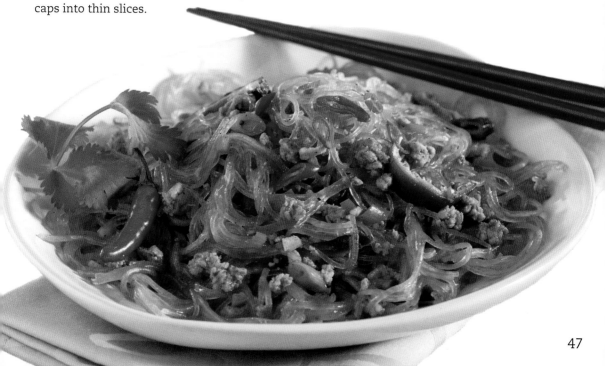

Cereal

This standard breakfast item gets way more attention in a gluten-free diet. Corn and rice cereals, in particular, go above and beyond the basic morning bowl with milk when used for snacks, treats, coatings and more.

Benefits

Because rice and corn cereals are not overly sweet, they have tons of nontraditional uses in a gluten-free kitchen. When crushed, they can be used on their own or combined with gluten-free flours and seasonings and used in place of bread crumbs for a coating for fish or chicken. They can also be used to replace the bread crumbs that are typically called for in meatball or meat loaf recipes. And of course, they are great for dessert in the classic rice cereal treat.

Selection and Storage

While most plain corn and rice cereals are gluten-free, be sure to read labels carefully, since even the most popular brands contain gluten. They have a long shelf life, so they deserve a permanent spot in the pantry at all times—especially since they have so many uses. Store whole or crushed cereal in an airtight container.

Preparation

To turn cereal into bread crumbs, just place it in a resealable food storage bag and coarsely crush it. You can do batches of this at a time so that you always have ready-made bread crumbs on hand. To make very fine crumbs, process cereal in a food processor. Feel free to add dried herbs or seasonings to the crumb mixture for extra flavor.

Recipe Suggestions

Make a snack mix using any combination of cereals, nuts, dried fruits and chocolate pieces. Pack it in small containers or plastic bags so that you can always count on having something to eat when your gluten-free options may be limited. Get creative with a basic rice cereal treat recipe and try adding other ingredients like chocolate chips, nuts and dried cranberries. Or try making rice cereal pops for a fun, party-pleasing treat everyone will love. Roll the cereal and marshmallow mixture into balls, insert lollipop sticks and let stand until the mixture is set. Then dip the pops into melted chocolate or colored candy coatings. You can get even more creative and roll the pops in nuts, coconut or sprinkles while the chocolate or coating is still wet.

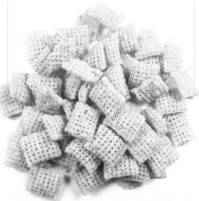

meat loaf cupcakes

- 3 medium potatoes, peeled and chopped
- 1½ pounds 90% lean ground beef
- ½ cup finely chopped onion
- ⅓ cup crushed gluten-free corn or rice cereal squares
- 1 egg
- 2 tablespoons chopped fresh rosemary leaves
- ½ cup whole milk
- 2 tablespoons margarine
- 1 teaspoon salt
- Black pepper
- ¼ cup snipped fresh chives

1. Preheat oven to 350°F. Place potatoes in medium saucepan; add enough water to cover. Bring to a boil; cook 25 to 30 minutes or until potatoes are fork-tender.

2. Meanwhile, combine beef, onion, cereal, egg and rosemary in large bowl; mix well. Divide mixture evenly among 10 standard (2½-inch) muffin cups or silicone baking cups. Bake 25 minutes or until cooked through (160°F).

3. Beat potatoes, milk, margarine, salt and pepper in large bowl with electric mixer at medium speed 3 minutes or until smooth. Place mashed potatoes in piping bag fitted with large star tip.

4. Remove meat loaf cupcakes to serving platter. Pipe mashed potatoes on top. Sprinkle with chives.

Makes 10 servings

nutrients per serving:

Calories 194
Calories from Fat 45%
Protein 16g
Carbohydrate 11g
Fiber 1g

Total Fat 9g
Saturated Fat 3g
Cholesterol 63mg
Sodium 327mg

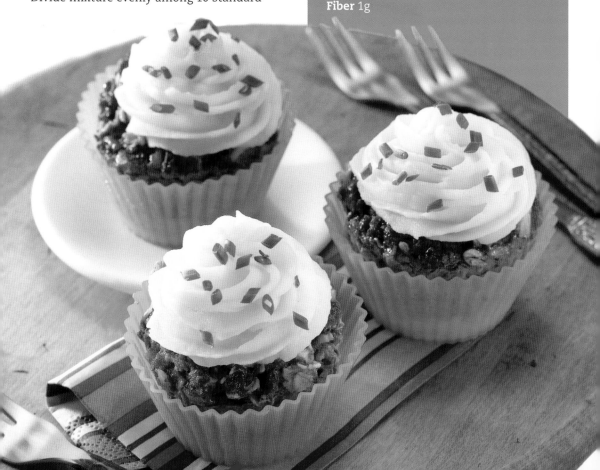

Cheese

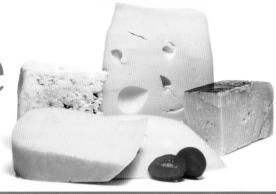

Benefits

Cheese is one of the few foods that gluten-free dieters can count on when eating out or eating on the run—and it's a nutritious option, too. A 1-ounce serving of most types of cheese is equivalent to one serving of high-quality protein, which makes cheese a satisfying food that staves off hunger. Even more, it is a concentrated source of many of the other nutrients found in milk, including calcium, phosphorus, magnesium, potassium, vitamin A, vitamin B$_{12}$ and riboflavin. One serving of cheese typically contains 20 percent of the recommended daily intake of calcium, an essential mineral that is necessary for building bone mass in children and young adults. And cheese helps fight tooth decay by protecting teeth from cavity-causing bacteria.

Selection and Storage

There are lots of varieties of cheese and many are available in various flavors and forms (sliced, cubed, shredded, grated, crumbled, in blocks, sticks and spreads). Cheese should be kept refrigerated. Packaged

There are hundreds of types of cheese available today, each with its own distinctive flavor and texture. While their uses in cooking may vary, they are all filled with protein and other important nutrients.

prepared cheese, like shredded or sliced cheese, can be left in the original wrapping, but bulk cheese should be wrapped tightly in plastic wrap.

Preparation

Be sure blocks of cheese are chilled before shredding or grating. However, serving cheese at room temperature brings out the best flavor. When cooking with cheese—for example in pasta dishes or for cheese sauces— use a low temperature and cook it slowly; high temperatures cause it to become rubbery.

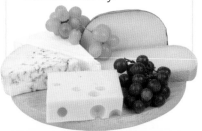

Recipe Suggestions

Any way you slice or shred it, cheese adds creaminess and a rich flavor that livens up any dish. Cheese pairs well with fruits, vegetables and grains, making these foods even more delicious. Try making a basic side dish with cheese, like broccoli in a Cheddar cheese sauce. Add some crumbled blue, feta or goat cheese to a green salad. Full-flavored hard cheeses, such as Parmesan or Asiago, or aromatic sharp cheeses, such as sharp Cheddar or Gorgonzola, should be used in smaller amounts because they have a more intense flavor. Small pieces of any hard cheese make great snacks, whether eaten on their own or paired with fruits and nuts.

creamy cheese and macaroni

1½ cups uncooked gluten-free elbow macaroni
1 cup chopped onion
1 cup chopped red or green bell pepper
¾ cup chopped celery
1 cup low-fat (1%) cottage cheese
1 cup (4 ounces) shredded Swiss cheese
2 ounces pasteurized process cheese product, cubed
½ cup whole milk
3 egg whites
3 tablespoons white rice flour
1 tablespoon margarine
¼ teaspoon black pepper
¼ teaspoon gluten-free hot pepper sauce

1. Preheat oven to 350°F. Spray 2-quart casserole with nonstick cooking spray.

2. Prepare macaroni according to package directions. During last 5 minutes of cooking, add onion, bell pepper and celery. Drain macaroni and vegetables.

3. Combine cottage cheese, Swiss cheese, cheese product, milk, egg whites, white rice flour, margarine, black pepper and hot pepper sauce in food processor or blender; process until smooth. Stir cheese mixture into macaroni and vegetables. Pour mixture into prepared casserole.

4. Bake 35 to 40 minutes or until golden brown. Let stand 10 minutes before serving. *Makes 6 to 8 servings*

nutrients per serving:

Calories 280
Calories from Fat 29%
Protein 15g
Carbohydrate 36g
Fiber 1g
Total Fat 8g
Saturated Fat 5g
Cholesterol 30mg
Sodium 380mg

Chicken

Because of its nutritional qualities, versatility and convenience, chicken has become a mainstay in the American diet.

Benefits

Chicken—especially chicken breast—is a staple because it is one of the leanest meats. It's a versatile source of high-quality protein with significantly less saturated fat than other types of meats. Chicken is also a good source of several B vitamins including vitamins B_6, B_{12} and niacin, which are important for healthy immune function. Furthermore, what makes chicken so great is that it can be cooked by a number of methods, and its mild taste is complemented by a wide variety of flavors.

Selection and Storage

Chicken is available in convenient, quick-cooking cuts like breasts, thighs, legs and wings. Breasts and thighs are available boneless and skinless as well as

bone-in and with skin. If buying preseasoned chicken, be sure to check labels to ensure any marinades or seasonings are free of gluten. Purchasing a whole chicken is an economical option. Whole chickens are available in sizes ranging from 2½ pounds (broiler-fryers) to 5 pounds (roasters). Refrigerate raw chicken for up to two days, cooked chicken up to three days. When freezing raw chicken, seal tightly in a plastic bag to prevent freezer burn. For best flavor and texture, use frozen chicken within two months.

Preparation

There are many cooking methods that can be applied to chicken. Whole chickens are usually roasted at 350°F. Both boneless and bone-in chicken parts can be broiled, poached, grilled, braised, baked, sautéed, pan-fried or stir-fried. It makes little difference whether the skin is removed before or after cooking, but the meat is more moist

and tender when cooked with the skin. Cook all chicken until the internal temperature is 165°F. Boneless pieces will cook faster than the bone-in parts; just avoid overcooking, which will make the meat dry and tough.

Recipe Suggestions

Since chicken has such a mild flavor, marinades and seasonings are welcome additions. Use any combination of flavors, savory or sweet, to add some great taste to your main course. Roast a whole chicken and use the meat for a number of meals. Serve some chicken with roasted vegetables for dinner and save some pieces to cut up and use in sandwiches or salads for lunch.

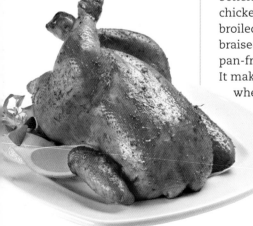

flourless fried chicken tenders

1½ cups chickpea flour
1½ teaspoons Italian seasoning
1 teaspoon salt
½ teaspoon black pepper
⅛ teaspoon ground red pepper
¾ cup plus 2 to 4 tablespoons water
  Vegetable oil
1 pound chicken tenders, cut in half
  if large
  Curry Mayo Dipping Sauce
    (recipe follows, optional)

1. Sift chickpea flour into medium bowl. Stir in Italian seasoning, salt, black pepper and red pepper. Gradually whisk in ¾ cup water until smooth. Whisk in additional water by tablespoons if necessary until batter is consistency of heavy cream.

2. Meanwhile, add oil to large heavy skillet or Dutch oven to ¾-inch depth. Heat over medium-high heat until oil registers 350°F on deep-fry thermometer or drop of batter placed in oil sizzles.

3. Pat chicken pieces dry. Dip chicken into batter with tongs; let excess fall back into bowl. Slide chicken gently into oil in batches. (Do not crowd pan.) Fry 2 to 3 minutes per side or until slightly browned and chicken is cooked through.

4. Drain chicken on paper towels. Serve warm with Curry Mayo Dipping Sauce, if desired.   *Makes 4 servings*

Curry Mayo Dipping Sauce: Combine ½ cup mayonnaise, ¼ cup sour cream and ½ teaspoon curry powder in small bowl. Stir in 2 tablespoons minced fresh cilantro.

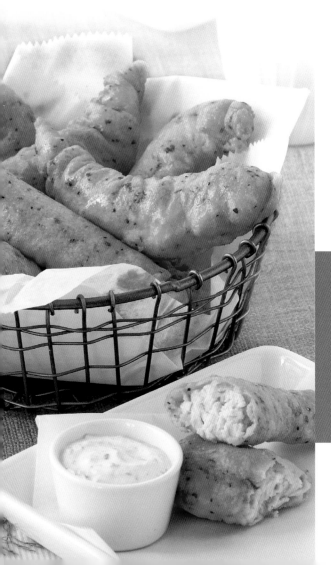

nutrients per serving:

Calories 372   **Total Fat** 17g
Calories from Fat 42% **Saturated Fat** 2g
Protein 32g   **Cholesterol** 59mg
Carbohydrate 20g   **Sodium** 860mg
Fiber 4g

Chickpeas

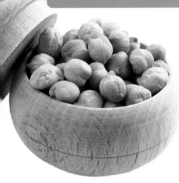

Chickpeas are a type of bean that deserves to be recognized for its many purposes in a gluten-free diet. These round, irregular-shaped, tan beans are also known as garbanzo or ceci beans.

Benefits

Chickpeas have a firm texture with a mild, nutlike taste that lends itself well to many gluten-free dishes, from soups and stews to pastas and casseroles to salads, dips and spreads. They are inexpensive and easy to prepare, and good eaten hot or cold. They are full of important nutrients too, including fiber and protein. And they provide more iron than most other beans do.

Selection and Storage

Chickpeas are available dried or canned. Look for dried chickpeas in plastic bags or bulk containers. Look for beans that are plump and free of blemishes and avoid those that are discolored or shriveled. Sort through the beans to be sure there aren't any with tiny holes, which indicate bug infestation. Dried chickpeas can be stored in an airtight container and kept in a cool, dry place up to a year. Convenient canned chickpeas are readily available, too.

Preparation

While canned chickpeas are more commonly sought after, dried chickpeas are cheaper and relatively easy to prepare. Sort through dried chickpeas and rinse thoroughly. Place them in a large saucepan and cover with water. Let them soak overnight. Drain the chickpeas and return to the saucepan. Add whatever liquid your recipe calls for (typically water or broth); about 1 cup of dried chickpeas requires about 3 cups of cooking liquid. Bring the chickpeas and cooking liquid to a boil over high heat. Reduce the heat to low and cover and simmer for about 1 hour. Cooked chickpeas can be stored in the refrigerator for up to three days. If using canned chickpeas, be sure to rinse and drain them well before proceeding with recipe directions.

Recipe Suggestions

Chickpeas are popular in the Mediterranean region and are therefore found in many Middle Eastern dishes, including hummus, a mixture of mashed chickpeas, tahini (sesame seed paste), garlic, lemon juice and oil. Make your own hummus and enjoy it as a snack with some fresh vegetable sticks or use it as a condiment for sandwiches. Chickpeas provide a wonderful nutty flavor to any dish they are in—add them to salads, pasta dishes, soups and stews.

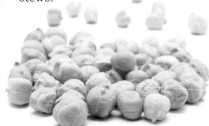

spicy roasted chickpeas

1 can (about 15 ounces) chickpeas,
   rinsed and drained
3 tablespoons olive oil
½ teaspoon salt
½ teaspoon black pepper
¾ to 1 tablespoon chili powder
⅛ to ¼ teaspoon ground red pepper
1 lime, cut into wedges

1. Preheat oven to 400°F.

2. Combine chickpeas, oil, salt and black pepper in large bowl. Spread in single layer on 15×10-inch jelly-roll pan.

3. Bake 15 minutes or until chickpeas begin to brown, shaking pan twice.

4. Sprinkle with chili powder and red pepper. Bake 5 minutes or until dark golden-red. Serve with lime wedges.   *Makes 4 (½-cup) servings*

nutrients per serving:

Calories 264
Calories from Fat 40%
Protein 7g
Carbohydrate 33g
Fiber 7g
Total Fat 12g
Saturated Fat 2g
Cholesterol 0mg
Sodium 730mg

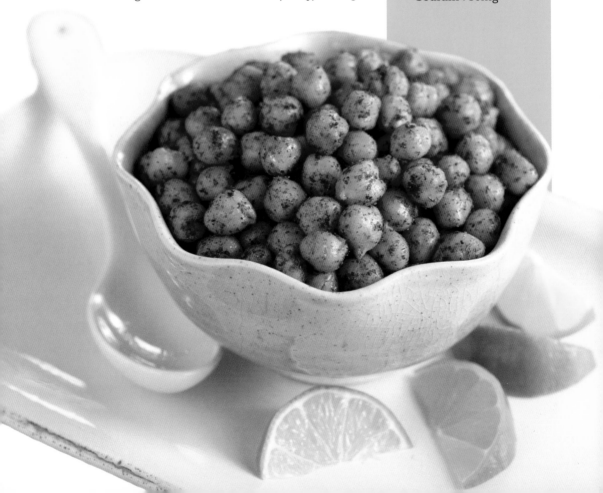

Chickpea Flour

Chickpea flour has been traditionally used in Middle Eastern cooking and baking, but it is now finding a new purpose as a gluten-free flour alternative.

Benefits

Chickpea flour is a hearty flour that is high in protein, fiber and calcium. Its high protein content gives it a great texture that works really well in baking, especially when combined with other gluten-free flour varieties. It can also be used as a thickening agent for soups, stews and sauces or as a coating for vegetables, chicken or fish.

Selection and Storage

Chickpea flour is used in many international cuisines and therefore may be found labeled differently, depending on the market. It is also known as garbanzo bean flour, channa flour, gram flour, besan flour and harina de garbanzo. While you may be able to find chickpea flour in the specialty food section of some supermarkets, you can also find it at Indian or Italian markets or order it online. If you do not plan on using chickpea flour right away, store it in the freezer for several months.

Preparation

Chickpea flour can be pricey, so you may want to create your own using inexpensive dried beans. Place dried chickpeas in a food processor or coffee grinder and process or grind them until they are finely ground and smooth. Be sure to sift the flour to remove any large pieces before using in any recipe—this applies to store-bought chickpea flour, too.

Recipe Suggestions

Chickpea flour has been used to add substance and nutrition to Indian cuisine for years—the rich flavor and texture complement traditional Indian spices well. Besides its use in Indian dishes, chickpea flour is also found in many Italian and Mediterranean recipes. It works great as a batter for fried chicken or crumb coating for vegetables, as well. To use as a nutty and delicious crumb coating, toast chickpea flour in a skillet for a few minutes before combining it with desired seasonings. You can also try adding a small amount of chickpea flour to gluten-free baking recipes for extra protein.

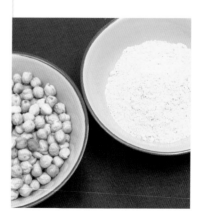

socca (niçoise chickpea pancake)

- **1 cup chickpea flour**
- **¾ teaspoon salt**
- **½ teaspoon black pepper**
- **1 cup water**
- **5 tablespoons olive oil, divided**
- **1½ teaspoons minced fresh basil** *or*
  - **½ teaspoon dried basil**
- **1 teaspoon minced fresh rosemary** *or*
  - **¼ teaspoon dried rosemary**
- **¼ teaspoon dried thyme**

1. Sift chickpea flour into medium bowl. Stir in salt and pepper. Gradually whisk in water until smooth. Stir in 2 tablespoons oil. Let stand at least 30 minutes.

2. Preheat oven to 450°F. Place 9- or 10-inch cast iron skillet in oven to heat.

3. Add basil, rosemary and thyme to batter; whisk until smooth. Carefully remove skillet from oven. Add 2 tablespoons oil to skillet, swirling to coat pan evenly. Immediately pour in batter.

4. Bake 12 to 15 minutes or until edge begins to pull away and center is firm. Remove from oven. Preheat broiler.

5. Brush with remaining 1 tablespoon oil. Broil 2 to 4 minutes or until dark brown in spots. Cut into wedges. Serve warm.

Makes 6 servings

Tip: Socca are pancakes made of chickpea flour and are commonly served in paper cones as a savory street food in the south of France, especially around Nice.

Note: Chickpea flour can also be used to make a thinner batter and cooked in a skillet to make a softer crêpe. Just increase the amount of water in the recipe by about ¼ cup.

nutrients per serving:

Calories 160	**Total Fat** 12g
Calories from Fat 69%	**Saturated Fat** 2g
Protein 3g	**Cholesterol** 0mg
Carbohydrate 9g	**Sodium** 302mg
Fiber 2g	

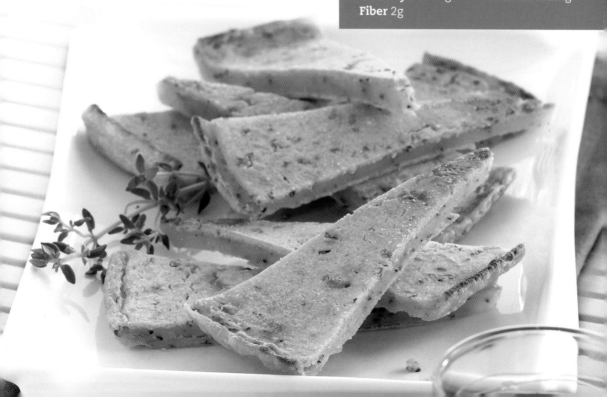

Chocolate

While it may seem too good to be true—it isn't! Lucky for those who have to avoid gluten, this decadent food can be a part of your diet.

Benefits

Chocolate is a best-loved food no matter how it is eaten—on its own, baked into sweet treats or melted into a sauce. Typically, unsweetened, bittersweet or semisweet chocolate is used in baking, while milk chocolate candies are enjoyed on their own. For gluten-free baked goods, chocolate provides a rich and smooth taste that often masks the undesired effects from using alternative flours—which is why so many gluten-free dessert recipes are chocolate based.

Selection and Storage

The quality of commercially available chocolate varies a great deal. Generally, higher quality chocolate has the best flavor. Make your selection based on your personal taste preference and intended use. Fine-quality chocolate breaks evenly, is smooth, not grainy, and has a shiny, unmarked surface. Since both heat and moisture adversely affect chocolate, it should be stored at room temperature, wrapped in foil or waxed paper, but not plastic wrap. Bittersweet and semisweet chocolate can be stored for several years, while milk chocolate has a much shorter shelf life and should be used within nine months.

Preparation

While adding chocolate chips or chunks to any dessert recipe is rather simple, melting chocolate can be more complex. It should be melted gently to prevent scorching. You can melt chopped chocolate or chocolate chips in a heavy saucepan over very low heat, stirring constantly. Be sure to remove the pan from heat immediately once it is melted. You can also melt it in a double boiler, which prevents scorching. The bottom pan should contain hot, but not boiling water, and the top pan with the chocolate should not touch the water. Make sure not to get any water whatsoever in the chocolate. Lastly, chocolate can be melted in the microwave, at about 60 seconds per ounce, stirring at 30-second intervals. However, this method can be tricky because if overheated, the chocolate will form clumps that cannot be remelted.

Recipe Suggestions

Chocolate is always enjoyed on its own but adds a decadent taste and texture to any dessert. Drizzle melted chocolate over cookies, cakes and even fruit. Make a chocolate fondue and serve with gluten-free cookies, cakes or fruit for an impressive dessert for parties and get-togethers.

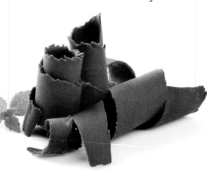

flourless dark chocolate cake

2 bars (8 ounces each) semisweet chocolate
½ cup (1 stick) butter
4 eggs, at room temperature, separated
¼ cup granulated sugar
2 tablespoons water
½ teaspoon vanilla
Whipped Cream (recipe follows)
½ cup raspberry jam

1. Preheat oven to 350°F. Spray 9-inch springform pan with nonstick cooking spray.

2. Melt chocolate and butter in medium saucepan over low heat; stir until well blended. Remove from heat. Add egg yolks, granulated sugar, water and vanilla; mix well.

3. Beat egg whites in large bowl with electric mixer at medium speed. Gradually increase speed to high; beat until stiff peaks form. Working in batches, fold in one third of chocolate mixture at a time until no white streaks remain. Pour batter into prepared pan; smooth top.

4. Bake 22 to 25 minutes or until center is set. Cool in pan on wire rack 30 minutes.

5. Meanwhile, prepare Whipped Cream. Place raspberry jam in small microwavable bowl; microwave on HIGH 30 seconds or until melted. Drizzle cake with jam and top with Whipped Cream.

Makes 8 to 10 servings

Whipped Cream: Beat 1 cup cold whipping cream and 2 tablespoons powdered sugar in large bowl with electric mixer at medium-high speed until soft peaks form.

nutrients per serving:

Calories 611
Calories from Fat 61%
Protein 8g
Carbohydrate 55g
Fiber 4g

Total Fat 43g
Saturated Fat 25g
Cholesterol 165mg
Sodium 55mg

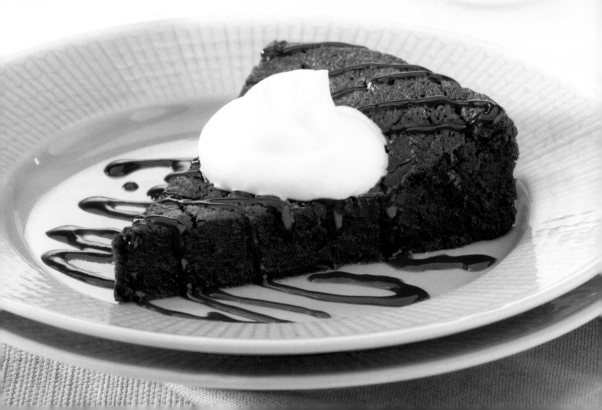

Cocoa Powder

This rich and flavorful powder is made by removing much of the fat, or cocoa butter, from the cocoa bean itself. It provides a wonderful chocolate taste and many health benefits.

Benefits

Cocoa powder is a concentrated source of plant nutrients called polyphenols, as well as minerals such as iron, magnesium, phosphorus, potassium and copper. Its antioxidant properties help stave off cancer and heart disease. Cocoa powder provides fiber, about 2 grams per tablespoon, and a small amount of protein. Using it is a great way to add a subtle chocolate flavor to foods.

Selection and Storage

Natural cocoa powder has a light brown color and is quite acidic, giving it a more bitter flavor. Alkalized cocoa powder, or Dutch process cocoa, has been treated to lower the acidity and has a richer brown color and more intense chocolate flavor. Keep cocoa powder in an opaque, airtight container in a cool, dark place for up to two years. Don't mistake cocoa powder for hot cocoa mix, which blends cocoa powder with powdered milk and sugar as well as many other additives that may contain gluten.

Preparation

Cocoa powder is most often used in baked goods such as cookies, brownies and cakes. When baking with cocoa powder, natural cocoa can create the rise in batter due to its high acid content, while Dutch process cocoa needs baking powder to create the same effect. Cocoa powder is also used for other treats, including puddings and beverages. To minimize lumps when using cocoa powder to make beverages or syrups, combine it first with the amount of sugar listed in the recipe before adding the liquid.

Recipe Suggestions

Cocoa powder is most often used in baking and may be used in place of unsweetened chocolate in recipes. For every ounce of unsweetened chocolate, substitute 3 tablespoons unsweetened cocoa powder plus 1 tablespoon butter. Cocoa powder has savory abilities, too, as in classic Mexican moles. It is even the "secret" ingredient found in many homemade chili recipes.

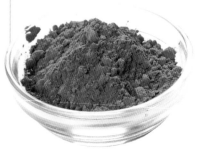
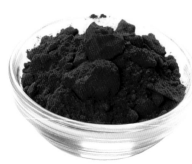

gluten-free caramel chocolate tart

Crust

- ¾ cup Gluten-Free All-Purpose Flour Blend (page 5),* plus additional for work surface
- ¾ cup unsweetened cocoa powder
- ½ cup (1 stick) cold butter, cubed
- 3 tablespoons sugar
- ½ teaspoon xanthan gum
- ⅛ teaspoon salt
- 3 tablespoons whipping cream
- 1 egg
- 1 egg yolk

Filling

- 1 cup sugar
- ¼ cup water
- 2 tablespoons light corn syrup
- 5 tablespoons butter
- ¼ cup whipping cream
- 1 teaspoon vanilla

Ganache

- ½ cup plus 1 tablespoon whipping cream
- 4 ounces bittersweet chocolate, chopped
  Raspberries (optional)

Or use any all-purpose gluten-free flour blend that does not contain xanthan gum.

1. For crust, beat ¾ cup flour blend, cocoa, ½ cup butter, 3 tablespoons sugar, xanthan gum and salt in large bowl with electric mixer at medium speed until mixture resembles coarse crumbs. Beat in 3 tablespoons cream, egg and egg yolk just until combined. Wrap in plastic wrap; refrigerate at least 1 hour or up to 3 days.

2. Roll dough on floured surface into 10-inch circle, about ¼ inch thick. Press into 9-inch tart pan. Trim edges to fit pan. Prick bottom with fork. Cover and refrigerate 30 minutes.

3. Preheat oven to 350°F. Line tart shell with foil and fill with pie weights or dried beans. Bake 15 minutes.

4. Remove foil and weights. Bake 10 to 12 minutes. Remove to wire rack; cool completely.

5. For filling, combine 1 cup sugar, water and corn syrup in large saucepan; cook and stir over medium-high heat until sugar is completely melted and deep amber color. Remove from heat.

6. Whisk in 5 tablespoons butter, ¼ cup cream and vanilla. Let stand 5 minutes to cool slightly. Pour into cooled crust. Let stand 45 minutes or until set.

7. For ganache, place ½ cup plus 1 tablespoon cream in small saucepan; bring to a simmer. Place chocolate in large bowl. Whisk cream into chocolate until smooth and blended.

8. Pour ganache over filling, tilting pan to cover completely. Refrigerate 2 hours or until firm and set. Garnish with raspberries.

Makes 8 servings

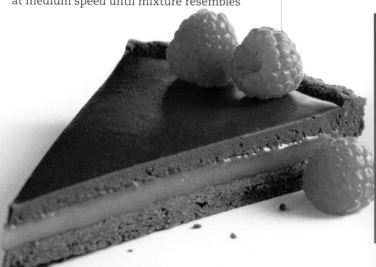

nutrients per serving:

Calories 548
Calories from Fat 58%
Protein 5g
Carbohydrate 55g
Fiber 3g
Total Fat 38g
Saturated Fat 22g
Cholesterol 137mg
Sodium 129mg

Coconut

This tropical fruit from the coconut palm adds flavor and texture to a wide variety of confections, desserts, salads and entrées.

Benefits

Coconut has a warm, sweet taste that is most often appreciated in baking. For gluten-free dieters, it provides not only wonderful flavor but a ton of moisture when used in dessert recipes. It makes a great garnish, too.

Selection and Storage

While fresh coconuts are available, more than likely you will be purchasing flaked or shredded sweetened coconut in plastic bags or cans. Find them in the baking aisle of the supermarket. Packaged unsweetened coconut is available at natural food stores. Unopened cans will last up to 18 months, while packaged sweetened coconut can be stored up to six months. Both should be refrigerated after opening or can be frozen for a prolonged shelf life.

Preparation

Toasting coconut really brings out its great flavor. To toast flaked coconut, spread it evenly into a thin layer on a baking sheet and bake in a 350°F oven for 5 to 7 minutes or until the flakes are a light golden brown color. Be sure to stir the coconut frequently to ensure even toasting. Tinting coconut is also a great way to add some color and décor to baked goods. Add a few drops of desired food coloring to 1 cup of flaked or shredded coconut in a small resealable plastic bag or bowl. Shake the bag or toss the coconut with the food coloring gently in the bowl until it is evenly colored.

Recipe Suggestions

Adding coconut as a garnish to desserts is common, but the best use of coconut in gluten-free baking is for classic coconut macaroons—a sweet treat that is made from flaked sweetened coconut, sugar and egg whites. Almost any desired ingredient can be added, from candies to nuts to chocolate. In fact, because this treat has no flour in it, it has always been enjoyed as a Passover dessert. Coconut also works wonderfully with main dishes, too. Try using flaked coconut as a coating for shrimp. Simply combine the coconut with desired seasonings and use to coat shrimp that has been dipped in melted butter. Bake in a 425°F oven for about 5 minutes and you have a wonderfully sweet and toasty meal.

homemade coconut meringues

- **3 egg whites**
- **¼ teaspoon cream of tartar**
- **⅛ teaspoon salt**
- **¾ cup sugar**
- **2¼ cups flaked coconut, toasted***
- **1 teaspoon vanilla**

To toast coconut, spread evenly on baking sheet. Bake in preheated 350°F oven 5 to 7 minutes or until light golden brown, stirring occasionally. Cool before using.

1. Preheat oven to 300°F. Line cookie sheets with parchment paper or foil.

2. Beat egg whites, cream of tartar and salt in large bowl with electric mixer at high speed until soft peaks form. Beat in sugar, 1 tablespoon at a time, until egg whites are stiff and shiny. Fold in coconut and vanilla. Drop dough by tablespoonfuls 2 inches apart onto prepared cookie sheets; flatten slightly.

3. Bake 18 to 22 minutes or until golden brown. Cool on cookie sheets 1 minute. Remove to wire racks; cool completely. Store in airtight container.

Makes 2 dozen meringues (3 meringues per serving)

nutrients per serving:

Calories 161
Calories from Fat 41%
Protein 2g
Carbohydrate 23g
Fiber 2g
Total Fat 8g
Saturated Fat 7g
Cholesterol 0mg
Sodium 62mg

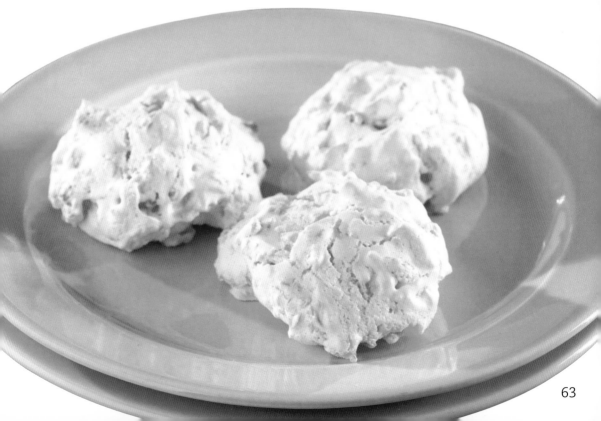

Coconut Flour

Coconut flour is a gluten-free flour alternative that provides subtle coconut fragrance and flavor as well as a natural sweetness whenever it is used.

Benefits

Coconut flour is a nutritious alternative gluten-free flour; it's high in fiber, a good source of protein and relatively lower in carbohydrates than other flours. In fact, the majority of the carbohydrate content in coconut flour comes from fiber, which aids in digestive health. Coconut flour is made from coconut meat that has been dried, defatted and finely ground. Because it is made from coconuts, it provides a unique, natural sweet flavor when used in baking.

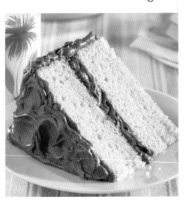

Coconut flour has a great absorbing capacity due to its high fiber content, so a little bit of this flour goes a long way.

Selection and Storage

Coconut flour can be found in the specialty flour section of many supermarkets and natural food stores. It can also be ordered online. Once a package is opened, store it in an airtight container in the refrigerator. If buying large amounts, freeze any flour that isn't going to be used right away in large resealable plastic food storage bags.

Preparation

When coconut flour is used alone in a recipe, it typically calls for less flour and more eggs than recipes usually do. This is because of the higher fiber content, which makes this flour more dense and heavier than other alternative flours. The eggs provide a necessary extra lift that helps prevent a heavy final product. Even though coconut flour provides a rich texture when used, it is a very fine powder, similar in consistency to wheat flour, and blends seamlessly with both wet and dry ingredients. It is a great thickener, too.

Recipe Suggestions

Coconut flour can be used instead of almond flour in the all-purpose flour blend in this book. This substitution is recommended for use in baking sweets and desserts because of the subtle sweet flavor it provides. Try it instead of almond flour in any cookie, bar or cake recipe in this book. Use a small amount of coconut flour to thicken soups, sauces or smoothies and you'll get extra fiber, too.

blueberry coconut flour muffins

- **6 eggs**
- **½ cup sugar**
- **¼ cup (½ stick) butter, melted**
- **¼ cup whole milk**
- **½ cup plus 2 teaspoons coconut flour, divided**
- **2 teaspoons grated lemon peel**
- **½ teaspoon salt**
- **½ teaspoon baking powder**
- **½ teaspoon xanthan gum**
- **1 cup blueberries**

1. Preheat oven to 375°F. Line 12 standard (2½-inch) muffin cups with paper baking cups.

2. Whisk eggs, sugar, butter and milk in medium bowl until well combined.

3. Mix ½ cup coconut flour, lemon peel, salt, baking powder and xanthan gum in medium bowl. Sift flour mixture into egg mixture. Whisk until batter is smooth.

4. Combine blueberries with remaining 2 teaspoons coconut flour in small bowl. Stir gently into batter. Pour evenly into prepared muffin cups.

5. Bake 12 to 15 minutes or until toothpick inserted into centers comes out clean. Cool in pan on wire rack 5 minutes. Remove from pan; serve warm. *Makes 12 muffins*

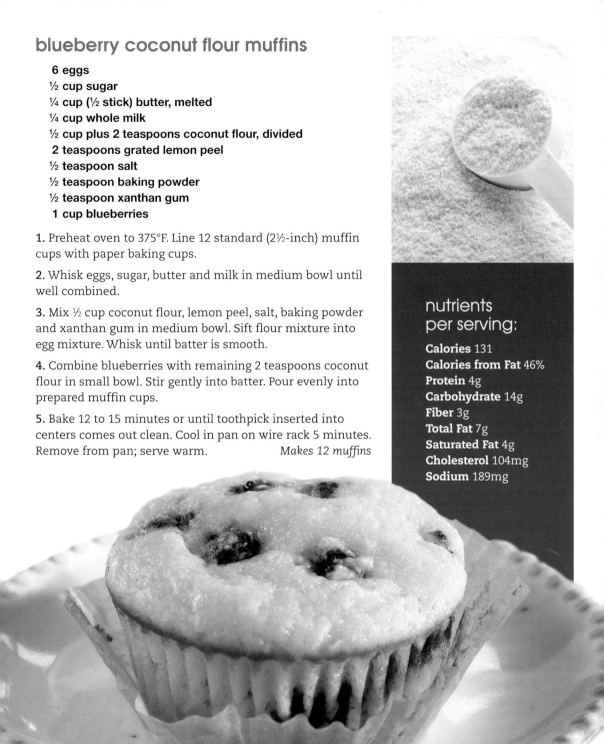

nutrients per serving:

Calories 131
Calories from Fat 46%
Protein 4g
Carbohydrate 14g
Fiber 3g
Total Fat 7g
Saturated Fat 4g
Cholesterol 104mg
Sodium 189mg

Corn Flour

Corn flour contains all the layers from the corn—the bran, the germ and the endosperm—making it a whole grain flour and an excellent addition to many gluten-free recipes.

Benefits

There may be some confusion when it comes to corn flour, as there are many different forms and varieties available, and luckily all are gluten-free. Regular corn flour is not the same as cornmeal, cornstarch or masa corn flour and works more like regular all-purpose flour. Cornmeal has a coarse, gritty texture and is denser than corn flour, which means that it works very differently, too. In fact, corn flour is merely a finely ground form of cornmeal. Cornstarch has been processed further and milled to an even finer powder due to the endosperm of the corn being removed.

Selection and Storage

Corn flour is relatively inexpensive compared to other gluten-free flours. It is regularly available in the supermarket near other flours or in the specialty food section. Be sure to purchase regular corn flour and not any other form of corn flour, including cornstarch, cornmeal, masa for arepas, instant corn flour for arepas, masarepa, masa al instante, harina precodica or masa harina.

Preparation

Corn flour is most commonly used in batters for fried foods, but it is a staple in a gluten-free pantry with even greater purposes. Corn flour has a soft, fine texture that is best used in making muffins, breads and tortillas. While it works in many recipes, it does have a subtle corn flavor, so keep this in mind when using. It can also be used as a thickening agent.

Recipe Suggestions

Use corn flour instead of cornmeal in muffins, breads, pancakes or biscuit recipes. It will produce a lighter, fluffier final product. You can also use corn flour as a coating for any fried food, from vegetables to meats and seafood—it produces a crispier breading than all-purpose flour does. Try using it to thicken any soup or dip recipe—just be sure the ingredients in the recipe go well with the light corn flavor the flour provides.

chewy corn bread cookies

- 1 cup (2 sticks) butter, softened
- ⅔ cup plus 2 tablespoons sugar, divided
- 1 egg
- 1 teaspoon vanilla
- ½ teaspoon salt
- 2 cups corn flour
- ½ cup instant polenta

1. Beat butter and ⅔ cup sugar in large bowl with electric mixer at medium-high speed until creamy. Beat in egg, vanilla and salt until well blended. Combine corn flour and polenta in medium bowl. Gradually add to butter mixture, beating well after each addition. (Dough will be very sticky.)

2. Shape dough into two discs. Wrap in plastic wrap; refrigerate at least 2 hours.

3. Preheat oven to 350°F. Line cookie sheets with parchment paper.

4. Shape dough into 1-inch balls. Roll in remaining 2 tablespoons sugar. Place 1 inch apart on prepared cookie sheets.

5. Bake 12 to 14 minutes. Cool completely on cookie sheets.

Makes 4 dozen cookies (2 cookies per serving)

nutrients per serving:

Calories 123
Calories from Fat 61%
Protein 1g
Carbohydrate 11g
Fiber 1g
Total Fat 8g
Saturated Fat 5g
Cholesterol 28mg
Sodium 5mg

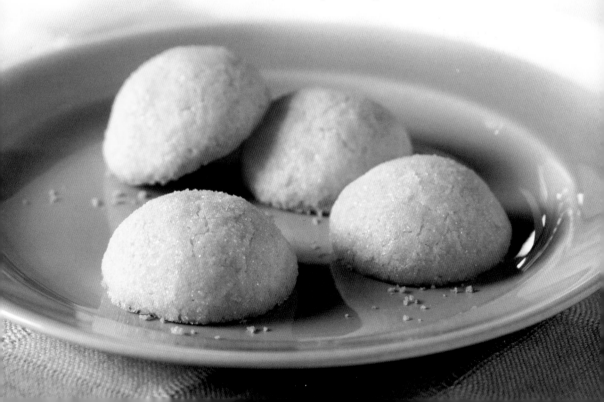

Cornmeal

Cornmeal comes in a variety of grinds and colors—from fine to coarse and white, yellow and even blue—and deserves a spot in any gluten-free pantry.

Benefits

Cornmeal gets its name from how it is made; it is the meal ground from dried corn kernels. It has a mild, nutty, sweet flavor that allows it to be used in numerous ways, though it's most often used in quick breads, as a coating and occasionally as a thickener. It is a staple in Italian kitchens because it is the base of the popular traditional dish polenta. There are two grades of cornmeal, fine and coarse. The fine grind is the most common and is more suited for baking into breads and muffins, but the coarse grind works better as a coating. While the most popular form is steel-ground cornmeal, look for stone-ground cornmeal, which contains the germ and hull of the corn and therefore has more vitamins and minerals.

Selection and Storage

Look for cornmeal near the flours at the supermarket. Pay attention to the grinding process and grade labeled on packages to be sure you are getting the product you want. Don't confuse cornmeal for instant polenta mix, which is made from cornmeal that has been precooked. If you purchase stone-ground cornmeal for its nutritious benefits, keep in mind it is more perishable. Store cornmeal in an airtight container in a cool, dry location for up to eight months or freeze it for up to two years.

Preparation

The coarse, gritty texture of cornmeal provides a natural crunchy bite whenever it is used raw, which is important to keep in mind when using it in recipes. Too coarse a grind can produce gritty baked goods. To get rid of the rough texture, be sure to purchase the fine grind and follow recipe directions, which will typically call to combine it with milk, broth and/or water.

Recipe Suggestions

The natural crisp texture is what makes cornmeal a great coating for fried or baked fish, meats or vegetables. Combine it with equal parts rice flour and any desired seasonings for an extra-crunchy finish. For a special side dish make polenta; its creamy, rich texture and mild taste work wonderfully with almost any food, from sautéed meats and vegetables to beans, cheese and herbs.

chili corn bread

Nonstick cooking spray
¼ cup chopped red bell pepper
¼ cup chopped green bell pepper
2 small jalapeño peppers,* minced
2 cloves garlic, minced
¾ cup corn
1½ cups yellow cornmeal
½ cup Gluten-Free All-Purpose
    Flour Blend (page 5)**
2 tablespoons sugar
2 teaspoons baking powder
1½ teaspoons xanthan gum
½ teaspoon baking soda
½ teaspoon salt
½ teaspoon ground cumin
1½ cups low-fat buttermilk
2 egg whites
1 egg
¼ cup (½ stick) butter, melted

*Jalapeño peppers can sting and irritate the skin, so wear rubber gloves when handling peppers and do not touch your eyes.

**Or use any all-purpose gluten-free flour blend that does not contain xanthan gum.

1. Preheat oven to 375°F. Spray 8-inch square baking pan with cooking spray.

2. Spray small skillet with cooking spray. Add bell peppers, jalapeño peppers and garlic; cook and stir over medium heat 3 to 4 minutes or until peppers are tender. Stir in corn; cook 1 to 2 minutes. Remove from heat.

3. Combine cornmeal, flour blend, sugar, baking powder, xanthan gum, baking soda, salt and cumin in large bowl. Add buttermilk, egg whites, egg and butter; mix until blended. Stir in corn mixture. Pour into prepared pan.

4. Bake 25 to 30 minutes or until golden brown. Cool completely in pan on wire rack.   *Makes 12 servings*

nutrients per serving:

Calories 152
Calories from Fat 33%
Protein 4g
Carbohydrate 22g
Fiber 2g
Total Fat 6g
Saturated Fat 3g
Cholesterol 27mg
Sodium 318mg

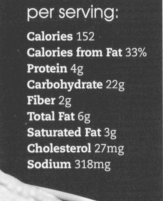

Cornstarch

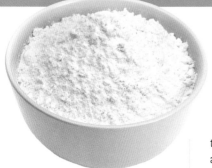

Cornstarch has probably always been a staple ingredient in your pantry, but it has even greater purposes than you might know.

Benefits

Cornstarch is a highly refined, smooth white powder made from the endosperm (center) of dried corn kernels. It is best used as a thickener, with about twice the thickening ability of flour. It also becomes clear when cooked while flour produces an opaque color. Traditionally, cornstarch has been used for stir-fries, sauces and puddings, but for gluten-free cooking, it can be used to thicken any dish, from soups, stews and casseroles to sweet treats like pie fillings, frostings and glazes. And its great thickening ability and bland flavor complements other gluten-free flours well for baking.

Selection and Storage

Cornstarch has the same thickening ability as other gluten-free thickeners, including potato starch, tapioca flour and arrowroot. However, cornstarch is much more widely available and significantly less expensive. You can find cornstarch in the baking aisle of the supermarket and even your local convenience store. Store it in an airtight container in a cool, dry location for several years.

Preparation

Cornstarch must be combined with liquid before using or it will produce lumps. Mix it with a cold liquid until smooth just before cooking or adding it to a hot liquid. In sweet sauces and puddings, mixing cornstarch with the granulated sugar in the recipe before adding the cold liquid will also prevent lumps. Cook any hot dish that calls for cornstarch over low to medium heat, stirring gently. Be sure not to overcook the dish or stir the mixture too vigorously, which will cause lumps to form and soups, sauces or other liquids to thin. It is important to note that cornstarch loses its thickening ability when frozen, so any sauce or liquid dish that uses cornstarch must be eaten soon after preparing.

Recipe Suggestions

Use cornstarch to thicken sauces and puddings. If you find a stew, soup or sauce recipe that calls for flour, use half the amount of cornstarch and be sure to mix it with liquid before adding it to the dish. Try any recipe in this book that calls for either gluten-free flour blend, both which contain cornstarch—including breads, muffins, cookies and other treats.

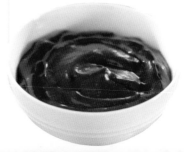

gluten-free apple pie

Gluten-Free Pie Crust (recipe follows)
6 medium apples, such as Gala, Jonathon
   or Granny Smith, peeled and cut into
   ¼-inch slices
¾ to 1 cup sugar, depending on sweetness
   of apples
½ cup dried cranberries
2 tablespoons cornstarch
2 teaspoons lemon juice
1 teaspoon ground cinnamon

1. Prepare Gluten-Free Pie Crust. Preheat oven to 425°F. Grease 9-inch pie pan.

2. Press one crust into prepared pan. Combine apples, sugar, cranberries, cornstarch, lemon juice and cinnamon in large bowl; toss gently. Arrange evenly in crust.

3. Place remaining crust over filling. Pinch edges of crust together; trim excess pastry. Cut slits in top of crust to allow steam to vent.

4. Bake 12 minutes. *Reduce oven temperature to 350°F.* Bake 30 to 40 minutes or until apples are tender when pierced with tip of sharp knife. Cool completely in pan on wire rack.

Makes 6 to 8 servings

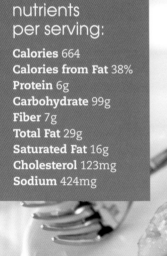

nutrients per serving:

Calories 664
Calories from Fat 38%
Protein 6g
Carbohydrate 99g
Fiber 7g
Total Fat 29g
Saturated Fat 16g
Cholesterol 123mg
Sodium 424mg

gluten-free pie crust

2 cups Gluten-Free All-Purpose Flour
   Blend (page 5),* plus additional for
   work surface
¼ cup sweet rice flour (mochiko)
1 tablespoon sugar
1 teaspoon xanthan gum
½ teaspoon salt
¾ cup (1½ sticks) cold butter
2 eggs
1½ tablespoons cider vinegar

*Or use any all-purpose gluten-free flour blend that does not contain xanthan gum.

1. Combine 2 cups flour blend, sweet rice flour, sugar, xanthan gum and salt in medium bowl. Cut in butter with pastry blender or two knives until mixture forms coarse crumbs.

2. Make a well in center of mixture. Add eggs and vinegar. Stir together just until dough forms. Divide dough in half; shape into two flat discs. Wrap in plastic wrap and refrigerate at least 45 minutes or until very cold.

3. Roll each piece of dough on floured surface to circle slightly larger than pie pan. (If dough becomes sticky, return to refrigerator until cold.) Wrap in plastic wrap and refrigerate until ready to use.

Makes 2 (9-inch) crusts

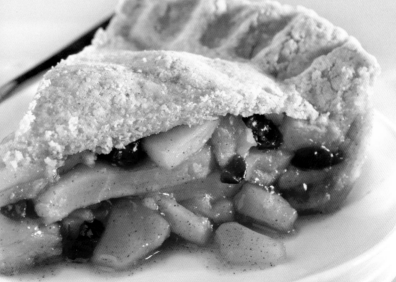

Corn Tortillas

Corn tortillas are the everyday bread of Mexico and a must-have for any gluten-free kitchen because they are so versatile.

Benefits

Living a gluten-free lifestyle requires a little creativity when it comes to meals, and corn tortillas are great for the number of ways they can be used. They can be wrapped, stacked, deep-fried or used to replace bread. They can be enjoyed with breakfast, lunch, dinner and even snacks. Their flexibility and multitude of uses make them an important food to keep on hand at all times.

Selection and Storage

When purchasing corn tortillas, be aware that some tortillas may be processed in a factory that also handles wheat products. It is also possible that corn tortillas have been dusted with regular flour to keep them separated from one another in the package— in this case, wheat should be listed as an ingredient. Make sure to always check labels carefully. While tortillas are often located in the bread aisle of the supermarket, traditional corn tortillas, which will not have any wheat added, can be found in the Mexican aisle. In some supermarkets traditional corn tortillas are kept in the refrigerated section near the cheese. They are best stored in sealed packages in the refrigerator or frozen for longer storage.

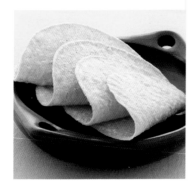

Preparation

Corn tortillas have a dry texture that may cause them to crack when rolled up. To warm tortillas to make them more pliable for use in wraps or sandwiches, wrap the tortillas in a lightly moistened paper towel and microwave on HIGH for 45 seconds to 1 minute.

You can bake your own tortilla chips, too. Cut each tortilla into six wedges and place them on a baking sheet. Add any desired seasonings and bake in a 400°F oven for 5 to 8 minutes or until crisp and brown.

Recipe Suggestions

Use corn tortillas to dip into soups and stews instead of bread or crackers, and try them for sandwiches and wraps. Their light sweet flavor and hearty texture work with any combination of vegetables, meats and cheeses. Try making some savory tortilla chips by brushing the wedges with a mixture of lime juice, ground red pepper and salt before baking. For a sweeter treat, brush the tortilla wedges with some melted butter and sprinkle with cinnamon and sugar.

Cottage Cheese

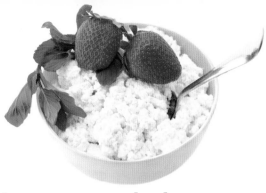

Cottage cheese has gotten a bad rap as a standard food in a weight-loss diet—but it is a wonder food for a gluten-free diet as an ingredient in many main dishes.

Benefits

Cottage cheese is a great base food for a variety of gluten-free dishes—it just requires a little creativity. Any fresh fruit or vegetables can accompany cottage cheese, so you can enjoy it for almost any meal— breakfast, lunch or even a snack. Plus, cottage cheese is rich in important nutrients, including a high protein count that fills you up, making it great for a satisfying meal. Cottage cheese also provides calcium and other nutrients found in milk but in lower

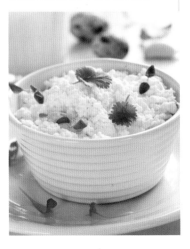

amounts, and it is lower in carbohydrates than milk and yogurt.

Selection and Storage

Choose low-fat (1%) or fat-free cottage cheese for less calories and fat than whole milk (4%) cottage cheese. It comes in small, medium or large curd, which does not affect its nutrition profile. While you can buy cottage cheese flavored, such as with chives or pineapple, it is best to buy the plain variety to ensure the product is gluten-free and to be able to use it in a variety of ways. Cottage cheese is perishable and must be stored in the refrigerator.

Preparation

The flavor of cottage cheese goes well with fresh vegetables or condiments, such as tomatoes, bell peppers and olives, or with fruits, such as pineapple, or berries. Cottage cheese is also a useful substitute ingredient for many higher-fat cheeses in various recipes from desserts to dips to casseroles.

Recipe Suggestions

Using cottage cheese as a base for a dish is so easy, it doesn't even require a recipe. You can simply make a sweet and satisfying parfait for breakfast by layering cottage cheese with your favorite fruits and nuts. For a fancy topping and extra flavor, add some toasted coconut and sprinkle with cinnamon and/or nutmeg. Use cottage cheese to replace cream cheese in dips or desserts such as cheesecake. Try substituting cottage cheese for the ricotta cheese in pasta dishes, like lasagna or stuffed shells. You can also use it in egg-based dishes, like quiches or frittatas, to replace higher-fat cheeses.

Dates

Benefits

While dates are very small, they are loaded with sweet taste and a ton of nutrients. Dates contain both types of dietary fiber—insoluble and soluble fiber—which play a role in keeping the very vulnerable digestive system of someone with celiac disease healthy. They are also high in potassium. While dates are valued for their important nutrients, they are even more appreciated for their use in baking. Dates have a much lower acid content compared to other fruits, which makes them work so well in baking by easily allowing doughs and batters to transform into light and fluffy breads, muffins and other treats.

Selection and Storage

You may not recognize fresh dates at first. They are oblong shaped with semi-firm textures and are dried, so their skins are somewhat wrinkled like raisins. There are many varieties, from plump and very soft to small and dry. The Mejdool date is available in the fall months and best eaten alone. The more common

What makes this fruit a key ingredient in gluten-free cooking—especially baking—is that it is a very concentrated source of sweetness that doesn't interfere with the way baked goods behave.

variety, the Deglet Noor, also comes fresh but is more commonly packaged whole, pitted or unpitted; they also come chopped in packages. Packaged dates are found near the other dried fruits in the supermarket. Store packaged dried dates in an airtight container at room temperature for up to six months or in the refrigerator up to a year. Fresh dates can be found in the produce aisle and should hold for up to a year well wrapped in the refrigerator.

Preparation

If you buy fresh whole dates, you will want to chill them before using. The colder they are, the easier they are to slice.

Recipe Suggestions

Dates are great on their own, but for a real treat, try stuffing them with nuts, such as whole almonds or chopped walnuts or pecans. Adding dates to breads, cakes, muffins and cookies adds richness and nutrients. Besides in baking, dates have a delightful taste that adds a sweet punch to savory dishes, too. Add chopped or slivered dates to your salad or stir them into your favorite coleslaw, chicken salad or tuna salad for a burst of flavor. They can also be enjoyed in meat and poultry dishes or side dishes, like rice pilafs or beans.

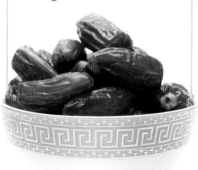

date & walnut bread

¾ cup chopped pitted dates
   (8 to 10 Medjool dates)
1 cup boiling water
½ cup brown rice flour
½ cup almond flour
½ cup cornstarch
¼ cup tapioca flour
¼ cup gluten-free oat flour
1 tablespoon baking powder
1 teaspoon xanthan gum
1 teaspoon baking soda
½ teaspoon salt
½ teaspoon ground cardamom
1 cup packed brown sugar
¼ cup canola oil
2 eggs
1 teaspoon vanilla
1 cup walnuts, coarsely chopped

1. Preheat oven to 350°F. Grease 9×5-inch loaf pan. Soak dates in boiling water in small bowl until dates are cooled and softened.

2. Combine brown rice flour, almond flour, cornstarch, tapioca flour, oat flour, baking powder, xanthan gum, baking soda, salt and cardamom in medium bowl.

3. Whisk brown sugar and oil in large bowl. Add eggs, one at a time, beating well after each addition. Gradually stir in dates with water and vanilla. Beat into flour mixture just until combined. Fold in walnuts. Pour into prepared pan.

4. Bake 50 to 55 minutes or until toothpick inserted into center comes out clean. (Check after 35 minutes and cover with foil to prevent overbrowning, if necessary.) Cool in pan 10 minutes. Remove to wire rack; cool completely.

Makes 12 servings

nutrients per serving:

Calories 305	**Total Fat** 15g
Calories from Fat 41%	**Saturated Fat** 1g
Protein 5g	**Cholesterol** 31mg
Carbohydrate 42g	**Sodium** 342mg
Fiber 3g	

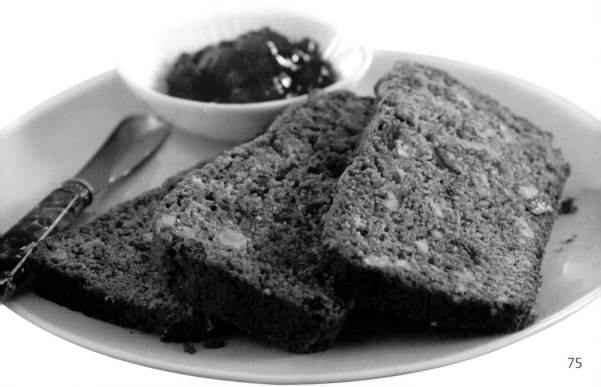

Eggplant

Eggplant is a very versatile and diverse vegetable and a common ingredient in many popular ethnic dishes, including Indian curries, Greek moussaka, Middle Eastern baba ghanoush and French ratatouille.

Benefits

Eggplant is an important ingredient in many dishes, from sauces and stews to dips and casseroles. The pale flesh, which becomes soft when cooked, has a mild, almost bland taste that combines well with many flavors. And eggplant's meaty texture makes it perfect for low-fat meatless dishes loaded with nutrient-rich grains, legumes and vegetables. Not only is eggplant low in calories and carbohydrates, but it is also is a decent source of fiber and potassium.

Selection and Storage

The most common purple-skinned globe variety is available year-round, with peak months of August and September. Choose eggplants that are small and firm, with unblemished, thin skins. Larger ones are seedy, tough and bitter. The skin should range in color from deep purple to light violet or white. Store eggplant unwashed in a cool, dry place. It is best used within a few days but may be refrigerated for up to a week.

Preparation

Eggplant can be eaten with or without the skin. Young eggplants have delicious, edible skin; older eggplants and white eggplants should be peeled. The easiest way to remove the skin is by using a potato peeler. Larger eggplants have a naturally bitter flavor that isn't always appreciated. To reduce this, slice the eggplant, sprinkle the slices with salt and let stand for 30 minutes; drain and blot dry before cooking. Eggplant can be baked, roasted, grilled, steamed or sautéed. It is fully cooked when it can be pierced easily with a fork.

Recipe Suggestions

Eggplant can be enjoyed in a variety of ways because of how adaptable the flavor and texture are. The meaty flesh of eggplant serves well as layers in casserole dishes, while its hearty shell serves as a great base for stuffing. You can't go wrong no matter how you enjoy it. Try stuffing eggplant with cooked grains, chopped veggies and cheese, and baking for a delightful, satisfying dinner. Eggplant also makes a tasty addition when diced and cooked in stir-fries, lasagna and pasta dishes.

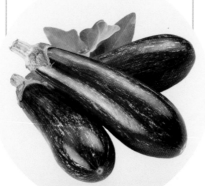

eggplant parmesan

- 2 egg whites
- 2 tablespoons water
- ½ cup crushed gluten-free rice cereal squares
- ¼ cup plus 2 tablespoons grated Parmesan cheese, divided
- 1 teaspoon Italian seasoning
- 1 large eggplant, peeled and cut into 12 round slices
- 2 teaspoons olive oil
- 1 small onion, diced
- 1 clove garlic, minced
- 2 cans (about 14 ounces each) diced tomatoes
- ½ teaspoon dried basil
- ½ teaspoon dried oregano
- ½ cup (2 ounces) shredded mozzarella cheese

1. Preheat oven to 350°F. Spray 15×10×1-inch jelly-roll pan with nonstick cooking spray.

2. Whisk egg whites and water in shallow dish. Combine crushed cereal, 2 tablespoons Parmesan cheese and Italian seasoning in another shallow dish. Dip eggplant slices in egg white mixture, then in cereal mixture, pressing lightly to adhere crumbs. Place in single layer in prepared pan.

3. Bake 25 to 30 minutes or until bottoms are browned. Turn slices over; bake 15 to 20 minutes or until well browned and tender.

4. Meanwhile, heat oil in medium nonstick skillet over medium-high heat. Add onion; cook and stir 5 minutes or until softened. Add garlic; cook and stir 1 minute. Stir in tomatoes, basil and oregano; bring to a boil. Reduce heat to low; simmer 15 to 20 minutes or until sauce is thickened, stirring occasionally.

5. Spray 13×9-inch baking dish with nonstick cooking spray. Spread sauce in dish. Arrange eggplant slices in single layer on top of sauce. Sprinkle with mozzarella cheese and remaining ¼ cup Parmesan cheese. Bake 15 to 20 minutes or until sauce is bubbly and cheese is melted. *Makes 4 servings*

Tip: For best results, cut eggplant into ½- to ¼-inch-thick slices.

nutrients per serving:

Calories 200
Calories from Fat 33%
Protein 12g
Carbohydrate 25g
Fiber 9g
Total Fat 8g
Saturated Fat 3g
Cholesterol 14mg
Sodium 781mg

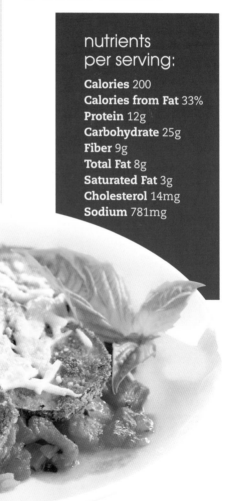

Eggs

Eggs are one of the world's most important foods. They can be prepared in many ways, however they are most notable for having several important functions in cooking and baking.

Benefits

For years, eggs have been shed in a negative light, yet they are actually quite incredible, being rich in many beneficial nutrients. Whole eggs offer 13 essential vitamins and minerals, high-quality protein, healthy unsaturated fats and protective antioxidants. And eggs have endless functions. They serve as an essential ingredient in recipes—helping baked goods to rise, binding ingredients in meat loaves, thickening custards and sauces and emulsifying mayonnaise and salad dressings. Egg whites are best used when whipped into a dessert topping or foam used to leaven cakes.

Selection and Storage

Select clean, unbroken grade AA or A eggs and refrigerate immediately after purchasing. For best flavor, use eggs within a week; however, they will hold up to three weeks. You can purchase liquid egg whites in refrigerated cartons. Some dessert recipes call for powdered egg whites, which are often labeled as "meringue powder" because they are perfect for whipping into a meringue.

Preparation

If you want to enjoy eggs on their own, cook eggs until the whites are completely coagulated and the yolks begin to thicken. Yolks should not be runny, but they should not be hard either. Cook slowly over gentle heat and serve immediately. For hard-cooked eggs, use eggs that are at least a week old because they will peel easier. Place them in a single layer in a saucepan and add enough cold water to cover by 1 inch. Cover and bring to a boil over high heat; remove from heat and let stand about 10 minutes. Pour off the hot water, cover with cold water and let stand until cooled. Crack the egg gently against a hard surface and peel.

Recipe Suggestions

Enjoy eggs for breakfast in an omelet with your favorite meats and vegetables, or create your own hash by sautéing some shredded potatoes with any other desired ingredients and topping with fried eggs. Hard-cooked eggs make the perfect gluten-free snack or breakfast on the go, as they are convenient, portable and satisfying. You can also use hard-cooked eggs to make egg salad, or chop or slice them and add to lettuce-based salads.

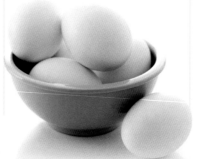

denver brunch bake

  2 tablespoons butter, divided
  ½ cup diced onion
  ½ cup diced green bell pepper
  ½ cup diced red bell pepper
  ½ cup cubed ham
  6 eggs
  1 cup whole milk
  ½ teaspoon salt
  ¼ teaspoon red pepper flakes
  4 slices gluten-free bread, cut into ½-inch cubes
  ¾ cup (3 ounces) shredded Cheddar cheese, divided

1. Grease 9-inch glass baking dish with 1 tablespoon butter.

2. Melt remaining 1 tablespoon butter in large nonstick skillet over medium heat. Add onion and bell peppers; cook and stir 3 minutes. Add ham; cook and stir 2 minutes. Remove from heat.

3. Beat eggs, milk, salt and red pepper flakes in large bowl. Add bread cubes, ham mixture and ½ cup cheese; mix well. Pour into prepared dish. Cover and refrigerate 8 hours or overnight.

4. Preheat oven to 350°F. Sprinkle egg mixture with remaining ¼ cup cheese.

5. Bake 45 minutes to 1 hour or until knife inserted into center comes out clean.   *Makes 4 servings*

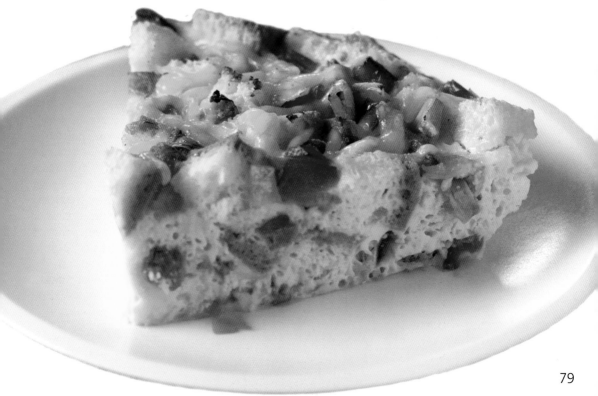

Fish

It's no surprise that fish is growing in popularity—it is versatile, delicious and nutritious. And it cooks quickly, making it perfect for weeknight meals.

Benefits

Fish is a smart choice in any diet, and luckily it is a food that is naturally gluten-free and can be prepared in many different ways. Fish contain omega-3 fatty acids, which are a form of healthy unsaturated fats that have been shown to help prevent heart disease and cancer, treat arthritis, reduce inflammation and depression and improve memory. Some fish are considered "fatty" because they have more omega-3 fats, including salmon, mackerel, herring, sardines, anchovies and trout. Leaner fish also provide some omega-3s, including tuna, whitefish, bass, ocean perch and halibut.

Selection and Storage

Fish can be purchased whole or as fillets or steaks at any supermarket. For whole fish, the skin should be moist and shiny with firm flesh. Fillets and steaks should have moist flesh that is free from discoloration and skin that is shiny. When storing fresh fish, wrap it tightly in plastic wrap, store in the coldest part of the refrigerator and use within a day. For extra convenience, frozen fish fillets are also readily available.

Preparation

For leaner fish (typically varieties with light-colored flesh), use moist-heat methods, such as poaching, steaming or baking. Dry-heat methods, such as baking, broiling

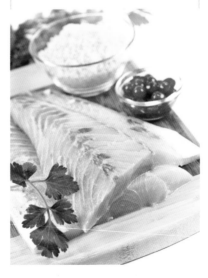

and grilling, work well for fattier fish. Fish cooks quite fast; it's done when it looks opaque and the flesh just begins to flake when tested with a fork. The rule of thumb is to bake for 8 to 10 minutes per inch of thickness, measured at the thickest point. For grilling or broiling, cook for 4 to 5 minutes per inch of thickness.

Recipe Suggestions

Many at-home chefs are apprehensive when it comes to purchasing and preparing fish and only enjoy it at restaurants, but there are so many quick and easy ways to prepare it. Make fish the main part of your meal. Whitefish has a mild taste that adapts to almost any flavor; try baking it with some lemon juice and a combination of your favorite Greek or Italian seasonings. For a crunchy fillet, crush some corn or rice cereal and combine the crumbs with garlic powder, salt and pepper and use as bread crumbs.

fish and "chips"

3 cups gluten-free crisp rice cereal, divided
1 egg
1 tablespoon water
1 pound cod, haddock or other firm white fish fillets
1½ teaspoons Italian seasoning, divided
Salt and black pepper
2 tablespoons butter, melted
2 medium zucchini, cut into sticks
1 package (8 ounces) carrot sticks
1 tablespoon olive oil

1. Preheat oven to 350°F. Spray baking sheet with nonstick cooking spray or line with foil.

2. Place 2 cups cereal in resealable food storage bag; coarsely crush with rolling pin. Combine with remaining 1 cup cereal in large shallow dish. Beat egg and water in separate shallow dish.

3. Cut fish into pieces, 3 to 4 inches long and about 2 inches wide. Sprinkle with 1 teaspoon Italian seasoning. Season with salt and pepper. Dip in egg, turning to coat all sides. Dip in cereal, turning to coat all sides. Place on prepared baking sheet. Drizzle with butter.

4. Place zucchini and carrot sticks on same baking sheet in single layer. Drizzle with oil and sprinkle with remaining ½ teaspoon Italian seasoning. Season with salt and pepper.

5. Bake 20 to 25 minutes or until fish is opaque in center and vegetables are tender.   *Makes 4 servings*

nutrients per serving:

Calories 310
Calories from Fat 34%
Protein 25g
Carbohydrate 27g
Fiber 3g
Total Fat 12g
Saturated Fat 5g
Cholesterol 110mg
Sodium 355mg

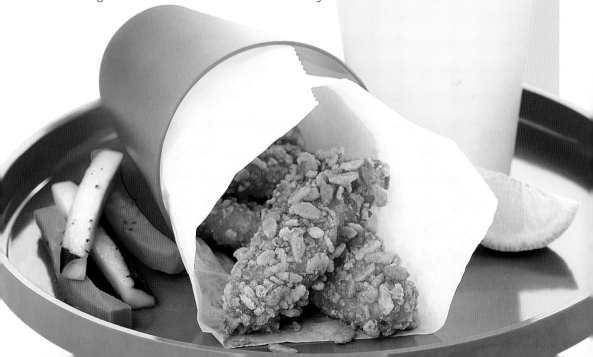

Gelatin

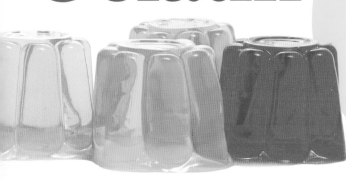

Most commonly known for its use in molded, fruit-flavored desserts, gelatin gains more respect in the gluten-free world as an all-important ingredient for use in baking.

Benefits

Unflavored gelatin is a colorless and tasteless thickening agent that often gives body to chilled, molded salads and desserts, but it has new life when it is used in gluten-free baking. Many gluten-free bread recipes have difficulty gaining the same height and volume as regular bread recipes do. Gelatin powder can be used as a dry ingredient to increase the amount that the baked good will rise.

Selection and Storage

Unflavored gelatin powder most often comes in ¼-ounce envelopes that contain about 1 tablespoon. It is located in the baking aisle of the supermarket. Fruit-flavored sweetened dry gelatin packages are also readily available, but be sure to read ingredient labels carefully because they may have gluten-containing flavoring or additives.

Preparation

When using gelatin to bake yeast breads, quick breads or muffins, the dried powder can be added directly to the batter. When using unflavored or flavored gelatin powders to make molds or mousses, the gelatin will need to be softened first. To soften, place ¼ cup of cold liquid (use whatever liquid the recipe calls for) in a small bowl or saucepan and evenly sprinkle with the gelatin powder. Let it stand about 5 minutes. To dissolve gelatin, place the bowl in a larger container of hot water and let it stand until all the crystals have dissolved. Softened gelatin can also be added to a hot mixture or heated in a saucepan over very low heat until dissolved. Be sure not to boil softened gelatin, or it will lose its thickening ability.

Recipe Suggestions

Besides its use in baking, gelatin is a great ingredient to keep on hand for traditional purposes, too—gelatin molds are a refreshing and enjoyable gluten-free treat. Make a gelatin salad using any combination of your favorite fruits and juices. Or use it to make a rich-tasting mousse using your favorite type of chocolate and cream or milk. Keep in mind that a ¼-ounce envelope of unflavored gelatin, or 1 tablespoon of granulated powder, will gel about 2 cups of most liquids.

rosemary bread

- 2½ cups Gluten-Free Flour Blend for Breads (page 5), plus additional for pan
- 1 tablespoon active dry yeast
- 1 tablespoon chopped fresh rosemary leaves
- 1½ teaspoons xanthan gum
- 1 teaspoon unflavored gelatin
- ½ teaspoon salt
- 2 eggs
- ¼ cup extra virgin olive oil
- ¾ cup warm whole milk (110°F)*

Milk should be warm, but not over 120°F, which will kill yeast. Test temperature on inner wrist. Milk should feel warmer than body temperature, not burning hot.

1. Let all ingredients stand at room temperature before preparing recipe. Spray 8×4-inch loaf pan with nonstick cooking spray; dust with flour blend.

2. Combine 2½ cups flour blend, yeast, rosemary, xanthan gum, gelatin and salt in large bowl. Beat eggs and oil in small bowl.

3. Beat egg mixture and milk into flour mixture with electric mixer at low speed until combined. Beat at high speed 3 to 4 minutes. (Batter should be smooth and stretchy.)

4. Spoon batter into prepared pan. Level top with dampened fingers or oiled spoon. Cover loosely; let rise in warm place about 45 minutes or until batter comes within 1 inch of top of pan.

5. Preheat oven to 400°F.

6. Bake 10 minutes. *Reduce oven temperature to 350°F.* Cover bread loosely with foil. Bake 35 to 45 minutes or until bread sounds hollow when tapped and internal temperature is 190°F. Remove from pan; cool completely on wire rack.

Makes 12 servings

nutrients per serving:

Calories 159	**Total Fat** 6g
Calories from Fat 36%	**Saturated Fat** 1g
Protein 3g	**Cholesterol** 0mg
Carbohydrate 22g	**Sodium** 119mg
Fiber 1g	

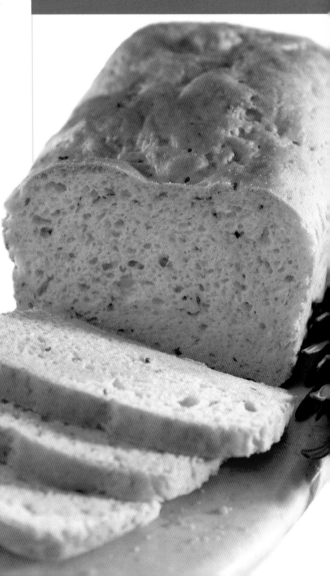

Greens

Greens often refer to a number of pungently flavored dark green leaves including, but not limited to, collard greens, Dandelion greens, mustard greens, beet greens, turnip greens, Swiss chard and kale.

Benefits

All types of green leafy vegetables have been gaining attention over the past few years in the nutrition and culinary worlds, and as a result are becoming more available at supermarkets and restaurants. Generally, all are good sources of various nutrients, particularly beta-carotene (a form of vitamin A), vitamin C, iron and calcium.

Selection and Storage

All greens should be chosen for their crisp, bright and evenly colored leaves. Avoid greens that are wilted, yellowed, spotted or have thick, fibrous stems. Store all greens in plastic bags in the refrigerator. Depending on the variety, they will last from three days to almost a week.

Preparation

Most greens can be eaten raw if they are young and tender, but they are more commonly enjoyed cooked when they are mature to enhance their flavor. Cooking greens also reduces the natural bitter flavor that accompanies greens. To cook them, soak them in a large bowl of cool water to remove any sand or dirt. Some varieties, like collard greens, have tough stems that should be removed. Simply pull the stem toward the top of the leaf and discard. All

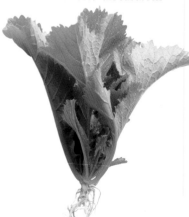

greens can be blanched, braised, sautéed, simmered, steamed or stir-fried.

Recipe Suggestions

No matter what type of greens you enjoy, you can't go wrong. They are most often cooked and served as a side dish. Create your own savory side dish by combining sautéed greens with onion, mushrooms, some diced bacon or ham and a splash of vinegar. Green leafy vegetables can easily be added to mixed dishes like hearty stews or casseroles because their taste blends well with other highly flavored ingredients. You can also add any variety of chopped greens to soups, stews and stir-fries. You may enjoy eating greens raw. Swap some chopped kale for lettuce in a salad for a stronger flavor, bite and extra nutrients. Top it with some citrus fruits, sliced almonds and a sweet vinaigrette dressing.

kale chips

1 large bunch kale (about 1 pound)
1 to 2 tablespoons olive oil
1 teaspoon garlic salt or other seasoned salt

nutrients per serving:

Calories 43
Calories from Fat 49%
Protein 2g
Carbohydrate 5g
Fiber 1g
Total Fat 3g
Saturated Fat <1g
Cholesterol 0mg
Sodium 180mg

1. Preheat oven to 350°F. Line baking sheets with parchment paper.

2. Wash kale and pat dry with paper towels. Remove center ribs and stems; discard. Cut leaves into 2- to 3-inch-wide pieces.

3. Combine leaves, oil and garlic salt in large bowl; toss to coat. Spread onto prepared baking sheets.

4. Bake 10 to 15 minutes or until edges are lightly browned and leaves are crisp.* Cool completely on baking sheets. Store in airtight container.   *Makes 6 servings*

If the leaves are lightly browned but not crisp, turn oven off and let chips stand in oven until crisp, about 10 minutes. Do not keep the oven on as the chips will burn easily.

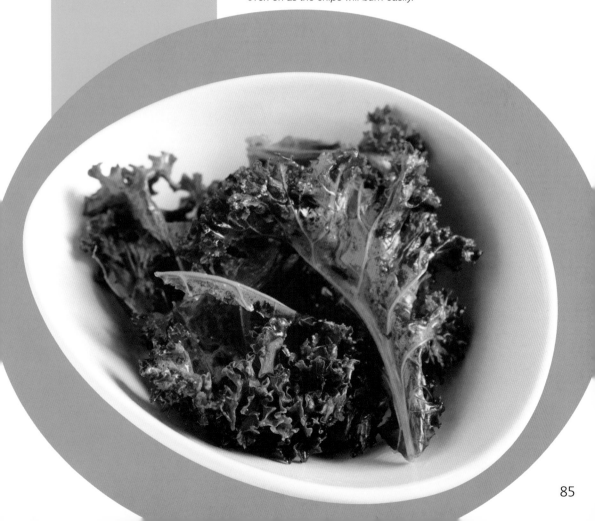

Grits

A popular Southern breakfast dish gets a new life in a gluten-free kitchen as a creamy dish that can be enjoyed any time of the day because it pairs well with almost anything.

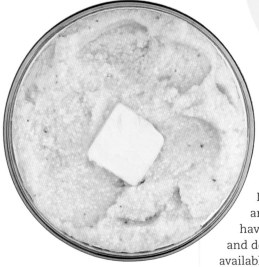

this gives them a coarser texture that is not always appreciated.

Instant grits, which are regular grits that have been precooked and dehydrated, are also available.

Benefits

Grits, also known as hominy grits, are a cereal made of dried, milled white or yellow corn kernels. They are often confused with another popular gluten-free dish, polenta, which is different because it is made from cornmeal. Grits have a light, sweet flavor that allows them to be prepared in many ways. There are different types of grits available besides regular grits. Quick-cooking grits, which are finely ground, are the most popular option since they can be prepared in just minutes. Stone-ground grits are the more nutritious choice though, because they contain the germ layer of the corn and therefore the fiber. However,

Selection and Storage

Quick-cooking and instant grits can be found near the other hot cereals in the supermarket. Stone-ground grits may be a little harder to find but should be available at natural food stores. Except for stone-ground grits, which should be refrigerated, grits should be stored in a tightly sealed container in a cool, dry place.

Preparation

Regular grits are cooked in liquid, usually water, milk or cream, in a saucepan over low heat and stirred frequently until the grits

are tender and all of the liquid is absorbed. Regular grits take 20 to 30 minutes to cook and require about 1½ cups of liquid per ½ cup. Quick-cooking grits cook in much less time, about 5 minutes, and require about 2 cups of liquid per ½ cup. For instant grits, follow package directions.

Recipe Suggestions

For a sweet and creamy breakfast, serve grits traditionally as hot cereal—either plain, with a pat of butter or a drizzle of maple syrup. Grits also pair well with cheese. Create a tasty side dish to accompany virtually any type of meat, poultry or seafood. Stir in your favorite type of cheese, sautéed onion, garlic and any other savory ingredients. Try using chicken broth instead of water, milk or cream to cook the grits for a boost of flavor.

shrimp and garlic-parmesan grits

2¼ cups water
½ cup quick-cooking grits
1 teaspoon dried oregano
½ teaspoon paprika
½ teaspoon dried basil
½ teaspoon salt, divided
¼ to ½ teaspoon black pepper
⅛ to ¼ teaspoon ground red pepper
    (optional)
1 tablespoon olive oil
8 ounces medium raw shrimp, peeled
    and deveined
¾ cup chopped green onions
2 tablespoons whole milk
2 tablespoons margarine
¼ teaspoon garlic powder
¼ cup grated Parmesan cheese
    Lemon wedges (optional)

1. Bring water to a boil in medium saucepan over high heat. Gradually stir in grits; reduce heat. Cover and simmer 9 minutes or until thickened, stirring occasionally. Set aside.

2. Meanwhile, combine oregano, paprika, basil, ¼ teaspoon salt, black pepper and ground red pepper, if desired, in small bowl.

3. Heat oil in large nonstick skillet over medium-high heat. Add shrimp; sprinkle with seasoning mixture. Cook 4 minutes or until shrimp are pink and opaque, stirring frequently. Remove from heat; stir in green onions. Cover to keep warm; set aside.

4. Whisk milk, margarine, garlic powder and remaining ¼ teaspoon salt into grits.

5. Spoon grits onto serving plates; sprinkle evenly with cheese and top with shrimp mixture. Serve with lemon wedges, if desired. *Makes 4 servings*

nutrients per serving:

Calories 192
Calories from Fat 54%
Protein 11g
Carbohydrate 11g
Fiber 1g
Total Fat 12g
Saturated Fat 3g
Cholesterol 77mg
Sodium 818mg

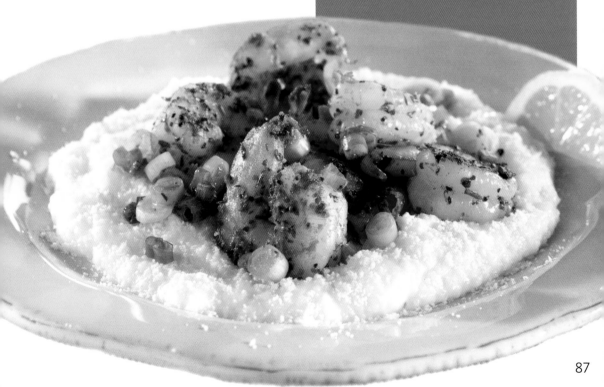

Gums

Xanthan gum and guar gum are the two most common gums used in gluten-free cooking. They are a helpful and often necessary addition to many recipes that lack gluten, especially baked goods.

Benefits

Gums are powders that help thicken and stabilize, and they are often added to commercial foods such as salad dressings, ice cream and low-fat dairy products. Used in gluten-free baking, they help bind, thicken and prevent the finished product from crumbling apart. Xanthan gum—made by fermenting corn sugar—is called for in most recipes for baked goods, from cookies, bars, muffins and cakes to pizza dough, quick breads and yeast breads. Guar gum—from the seed of a legume-related plant—may also be used in these instances, but it is most useful in cold foods such as ice cream, pudding and salad dressing.

Selection and Storage

Xanthan and guar gum can be found in the specialty baking section of natural food stores or ordered online. They are usually sold in small plastic packages, although guar gum sometimes comes in plastic bottles like large pill bottles. Xanthan gum is more expensive than guar gum. Store both in a cool, dry place or in the refrigerator for longer storage.

Preparation

Some prepared gluten-free flour blends already contain xanthan or guar gum, while many homemade mixes (including the ones in this book) do not, but instead call for it separately in the ingredient list. It is important to note this distinction because you do not want to unknowingly omit or double the amount of gum in a recipe. If you use too little, your baked goods will likely fall apart, and if you use too much, they will be heavy and gummy.

Recipe Suggestions

If you are new to gluten-free baking, you might want to just follow recipes that already include xanthan or guar gum. If you are more experienced and feel confident, you can try to adapt recipes on your own to include either gum. At times both gums can be used interchangeably, although you might need to use a little bit more guar gum than xanthan gum. In any case, you will only be using a small amount of either, usually from ½ to 2 teaspoons per cup of flour.

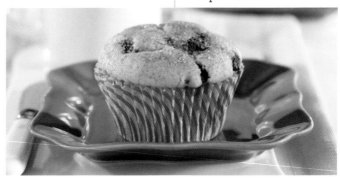

white chocolate pudding with crunchy toffee topping

¼ cup sugar
1¾ teaspoons guar gum
¼ teaspoon salt
2 cups reduced-fat (2%) milk
¾ cup whipping cream
7 squares (1 ounce each) white chocolate, chopped
2 teaspoons vanilla
    Crunchy Toffee Topping (recipe follows)

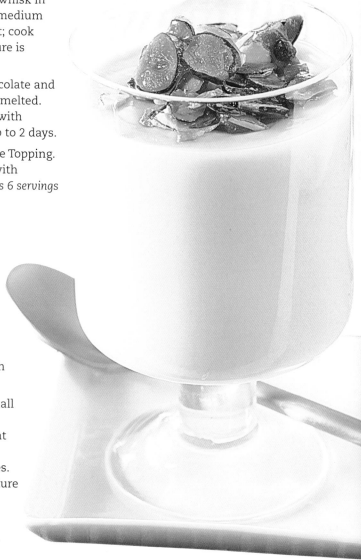

1. Combine sugar, guar gum and salt in medium saucepan; mix well. Slowly whisk in milk and cream. Bring to a boil over medium heat, stirring constantly. Reduce heat; cook and stir 2 to 3 minutes or until mixture is thickened.

2. Remove pan from heat; stir in chocolate and vanilla until chocolate is completely melted. Spoon into six dessert dishes; cover with plastic wrap. Refrigerate 1 hour or up to 2 days.

3. Meanwhile, prepare Crunchy Toffee Topping. Just before serving, sprinkle evenly with topping. *Makes 6 servings*

crunchy toffee topping

½ cup sugar
¼ cup light corn syrup
1 cup sliced almonds
2 teaspoons butter
½ teaspoon baking soda
½ teaspoon vanilla

Microwave Directions

1. Spray 10×10-inch sheet of foil with nonstick cooking spray.

2. Whisk sugar and corn syrup in small microwavable bowl. Microwave on HIGH 4 minutes. (Mixture will be light brown in color.) Stir in almonds and butter; microwave on HIGH 2 minutes. Stir in baking soda and vanilla. (Mixture will foam.)

3. Spread mixture in thin layer on prepared foil; cool completely. Break into pieces.

Honey

Honey is one of the oldest sweeteners. Today it is most popularly used as a sweetener for tea, a spread for toast or biscuits or as an ingredient in baked goods—something that is much appreciated in the gluten-free world.

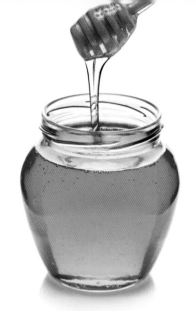

Benefits

Gluten-free baking can be rather challenging. Typically, breads, muffins and other sweets that lack gluten do not have a pleasant texture—they are often grainy or gummy. Honey is an important ingredient that not only provides a delicious natural sweet taste but also produces a better product with greater texture. Using honey for gluten-free baked goods results in a moist, dense product. Honey is an all-around useful ingredient that should be a staple on your pantry shelf anyway because it has so many uses besides baking.

Selection and Storage

While there are fresh forms of honey available in the market, the most commonly used honey is extracted liquid honey, which is made from the honeycomb and then heated, strained, filtered and often pasteurized. It is sold in jars or squeeze bottles near other condiments. Do not refrigerate honey, or it will become grainy and too thick to use. It can be stored for up to a year, tightly sealed, in a cool, dry place.

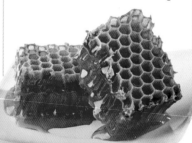

Preparation

Honey can easily be added to baking recipes, where it imparts a slightly sweet flavor with a distinct taste. In most cases, substituting honey for sugar in recipes is not recommended. Using honey in place of other liquid sweeteners, such as maple syrup, corn syrup and molasses, is usually successful.

Recipe Suggestions

You can use honey for so many types of dishes besides baked goods. Combine your favorite fruits and plain Greek yogurt and add a some honey for a morning smoothie that is sure to satisfy you. It also makes a great condiment and topping for many sweet and savory foods. Use it for a dipping sauce for sweet potato fries or chicken tenders, or drizzle it over a yogurt parfait or cottage cheese. It makes a great marinade, too: Combine honey with orange or lemon juice and use it for anything from salmon to pork chops.

Jicama

Often referred to as a Mexican potato, this easily overlooked root vegetable is refreshingly crisp and crunchy with a sweet, nutty flavor and radish-like texture.

Benefits

Not only does jicama have a sweet flavor and crunchy bite, it's a super food, nutrition wise. Jicama is very low in calories and an excellent source of vitamin C. It is also filled with fiber, a nutrient that is often lacking for people on a gluten-free diet because wheat is the main source of fiber for most Americans.

Selection and Storage

Jicama is available in most supermarkets from November through May. You may not recognize it at first; many think it resembles a large turnip. Jicama is round, large and has a tough brown skin. Select jicama that is firm and unblemished with a slightly silky sheen. It should not feel soft or appear to have bruises or wrinkles. Jicama can be stored for up to two weeks in a plastic bag in the refrigerator. You may also find jicama presliced and packaged in plastic containers near other prepared fruits and vegetables.

Preparation

The thin skin of jicama should be peeled before eating or cooking. Scrub the jicama with a vegetable brush under cold running water and peel off the skin with a paring knife. The layer near the skin may also need to be discarded, as it can often be tough and fibrous. Because it is difficult to prepare, it is best to cut the flesh of jicama into cubes or sticks when you get home from the supermarket so that you have it on hand to use whenever you want. Store cubes or sticks in an airtight container in the refrigerator.

Recipe Suggestions

Jicama is a versatile vegetable that adds a crisp bite and sweetness to foods. It tends to take on the flavors of foods that it accompanies, so the options for its use are limitless. However, its slightly sweet taste complements citrus flavors best. Add chopped or sliced jicama to any salad, salsa or coleslaw. It can also provide great flavor and texture to tuna or chicken salad. You can simply enjoy it alone as a snack or with a dip, such as guacamole. It can also be eaten cooked: Add jicama to stir-fries or soups during the last few minutes of cooking to retain its crispness.

Lentils

These legumes have a mild, earthy flavor and are versatile, inexpensive, easy to prepare and full of nutrients, so they make a great addition to any diet.

Benefits

Lentils are a wonderful meat substitute; they are loaded with satisfying protein and full of iron. They also supply a generous amount of other important nutrients. Lentils are high in fiber, which helps not only fill you up but also plays a significant role in digestive and heart health. Lentils are exceptionally high in folate—an essential nutrient for those with celiac disease because folate is often added to many gluten-containing processed foods like cereals and breads. Folate is important because it has been found to help prevent certain birth defects and may also help prevent heart disease and dementia.

Selection and Storage

Brown, green and red lentils are the most common varieties in the United States. You can purchase lentils in packages or bulk bins. Look for well-sealed bags with uniformly sized, brightly colored, disc-shaped lentils. If you buy them in bulk, watch for holes, which indicate insect infestation. When stored in a well-sealed container at room temperature, lentils keep for up to a year.

Preparation

Before using in recipes, sort through lentils, discarding any blemished ones or debris. Place the lentils in a colander and rinse with cold running water. Unlike dried beans, lentils do not need to be soaked before cooking. Combine lentils with water or broth in a saucepan— about 2 cups of liquid to each cup of lentils. Bring to a boil and then reduce the heat to low. Cover and simmer for 20 to 30 minutes or until they are tender.

Recipe Suggestions

Red lentils cook quickly and can become mushy, so they work best in creamy soups, purées or dips. Brown and green lentils retain their shape if not overcooked and are best served as a side dish or in salads. They pair well with chewy, hearty grains like brown rice. Lentils are willing recipients of flavorful herbs and spices, easily taking on the flavors of the foods they are mixed with. Use them in chilis, stews and soups or as a meat substitute for meat loaves, burgers or meatballs.

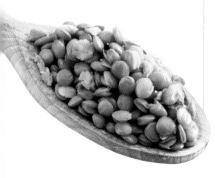

curried lentils with fruit

2 quarts water
1½ cups dried lentils, rinsed and sorted
1 Granny Smith apple, cored, peeled and chopped
¼ cup golden raisins
¼ cup lemon nonfat yogurt
1 teaspoon curry powder
1 teaspoon salt

1. Combine water and lentils in large saucepan; bring to a boil over high heat. Reduce heat to medium-low. Simmer 20 minutes, stirring occasionally.

2. Stir apple and raisins into saucepan; cook 10 minutes or until lentils are tender. Drain.

3. Place lentil mixture in large bowl. Stir in yogurt, curry powder and salt until well blended.   *Makes 6 servings*

Tip: Apples brown easily once they are cut. To prevent undesirable browning, sprinkle lemon, apple or grapefruit juice over apple pieces.

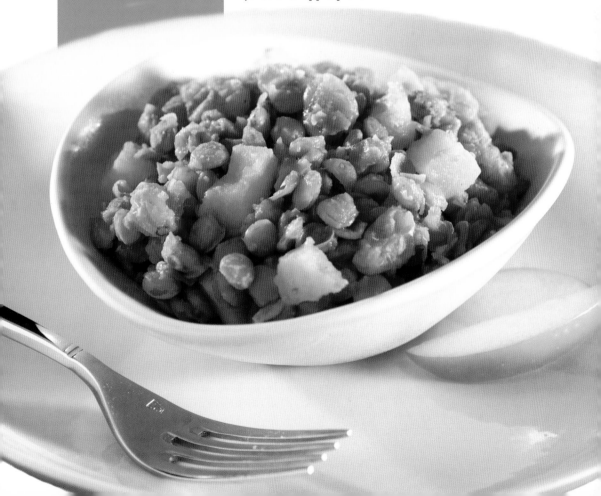

Lettuce

A staple in almost every diet, lettuce gains more appreciation in the gluten-free world for its many unconventional uses as a bread substitute.

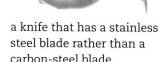

Benefits

Lettuce is so versatile, especially because there are so many varieties that range in color, texture and flavor. The best use besides a typical salad is for a bread or bun substitute for sandwiches, burgers and wraps. In fact, lettuce wraps can be requested at many restaurants. This is also a healthier option, as any type of lettuce is very low in calories. Some varieties are more nutritious than others, but they all are satisfying, versatile and filling. Lettuces that are dark green, including romaine, endive, escarole, looseleaf, butterhead, arugula and watercress, are the most nutritious. Generally speaking, the darker the color, the more nutrients it has.

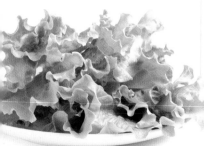

Selection and Storage

There are hundreds of varieties of lettuce, many available in your regular supermarket. Choose lettuce that is crisp and free of blemishes. If you purchase lettuce from a supermarket that periodically mists vegetables, dry the leaves before storing or add paper towels to bags of damp lettuce to absorb the moisture. Lettuce should be stored in an airtight bag or container in the refrigerator for three to five days. Prewashed, packaged salad greens are a convenient option.

Preparation

For heads of lettuce, remove the leaves and wash thoroughly under cold water, taking care to separate leaves so that any mud or grit will be rinsed off. Drain the leaves completely or blot with paper towels to remove excess moisture. To prevent browning, cut lettuce with a knife that has a stainless steel blade rather than a carbon-steel blade.

Recipe Suggestions

Get creative with a traditional lettuce-based salad. Combine lettuce with fresh fruits or vegetables, cold pasta, or chunks of chicken, turkey or tuna for a highly nutritious main dish. Add any favorite cheeses and toppings. For a crunch, use nuts or seeds instead of gluten-free croutons. When choosing salad dressing, be sure to read ingredient labels carefully for gluten-containing preservatives or additives. Or make your own dressing by combining flavored vinegar, citrus juice, olive oil and any desired spices and/or seasonings. For a lettuce wrap, use your favorite fillings, from Asian to Italian—lettuce has a mild flavor and light crunch that goes well with practically everything.

turkey lettuce wraps

- 1 teaspoon sesame oil
- 1 pound extra-lean ground turkey
- ½ cup sliced green onions
- 2 tablespoons minced fresh ginger
- 1 can (8 ounces) water chestnuts, chopped
- 1 teaspoon gluten-free light soy sauce
- ¼ cup chopped fresh cilantro
- 12 large lettuce leaves

Optional toppings

- Chopped mint leaves
- Chopped dry roasted peanuts

1. Heat oil in large skillet over medium-high heat. Add turkey, green onions and ginger; cook 7 minutes, stirring to break up meat.

2. Add water chestnuts and soy sauce to skillet; cook 3 minutes or until turkey is cooked through. Remove from heat; stir in cilantro.

3. Spoon ¼ cup turkey mixture into each lettuce leaf. Add desired toppings; roll up to enclose filling.

Makes 6 servings (2 wraps per serving)

nutrients per serving:

Calories 102
Calories from Fat 14%
Protein 18g
Carbohydrate 6g
Fiber 1g
Total Fat 2g
Saturated Fat <1g
Cholesterol 30mg
Sodium 87mg

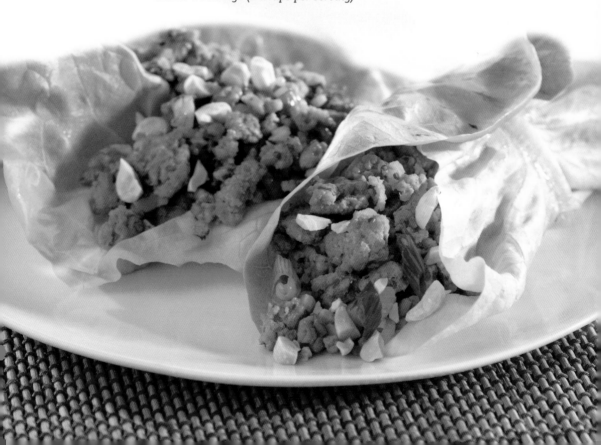

Maple Syrup

This flavorful, earthy sweetener is an excellent substitute for honey if you don't eat it or want some variety. It adds wonderful and unique taste to many sweet and savory dishes and is a must for pancakes.

Benefits

Maple syrup is made from boiling down the sap that is tapped from the maple tree. It is boiled down to varying degrees: Grade AA is light colored with a mild flavor; Grade A and B darken in color and deepen in flavor; Grade C is very dark with a strong, rich flavor. The grade you choose does not matter and is only up to personal preference. The best quality maple syrup and maple products come from Vermont, New York and Canada. Maple syrup contains minerals manganese and zinc, both important for immune function. In addition to having a higher concentration of minerals than honey, it also has fewer calories.

Selection and Storage

Maple syrup is sold year-round in all supermarkets. Smaller-batch, higher-quality maple syrup is often sold at specialty stores and some farmers' markets. Pure maple syrup is expensive, but the flavor is worth the splurge. Do not substitute pancake syrup, which is merely corn syrup that is artificially flavored. Keep maple syrup refrigerated after opening.

Preparation

Maple syrup is a wonderful ingredient for baked goods such as pies, cakes and other desserts. Use it when it is called for, and if you want to substitute it for honey, use ¾ cup maple syrup plus ½ cup granulated sugar for 1 cup of honey.

Recipe Suggestions

Maple syrup is the classic topper for pancakes and waffles. Also try it drizzled over hot cereal or yogurt. Use it to sweeten tea or coffee in place of sugar.

It is a wonderful sweetener for sweet potato dishes, from baked or mashed to casseroles to pies, especially when paired with warm winter spices. Use it as a glaze for meats, particularly ham, turkey and chicken. Make a dessert sauce to spoon over ice cream by cooking maple syrup with cinnamon sticks in a saucepan for a few minutes or until it thickens. Remove the cinnamon sticks and stir in a small amount of lemon juice.

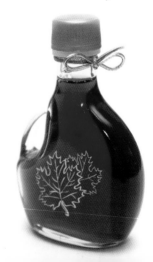

roasted chicken with maple glaze

1 **whole chicken (about 3 pounds)**
1 **onion, cut into wedges**
1 **orange, cut into wedges**
¾ **cup apple cider**
¼ **cup maple syrup**
¾ **teaspoon cornstarch**
¼ **teaspoon pumpkin pie spice**

1. Preheat oven to 325°F. Spray shallow roasting pan with nonstick cooking spray. Remove giblets and neck from chicken; discard or reserve for another use.

2. Place onion and orange wedges in cavity of chicken. Tie legs together with kitchen twine. Place on rack, breast side up, in prepared pan. Insert meat thermometer into thickest part of thigh, not touching bone.

3. Whisk apple cider, maple syrup, cornstarch and pumpkin pie spice in small saucepan until cornstarch is dissolved. Bring to a boil over medium heat, stirring constantly; cook 1 minute. Brush apple cider mixture over chicken.

4. Roast chicken 1½ hours or until meat thermometer registers 165°F, basting frequently with remaining cider mixture. (Do not baste during last 10 minutes of cooking.)

5. Discard any remaining cider mixture. Remove string from chicken; discard. Remove onion and orange wedges from chicken cavity; discard. Transfer chicken to serving platter. Let stand 10 minutes before carving.   *Makes 6 servings*

nutrients per serving:

Calories 317
Calories from Fat 52%
Protein 21g
Carbohydrate 14g
Fiber 1g
Total Fat 18g
Saturated Fat 5g
Cholesterol 87mg
Sodium 67mg

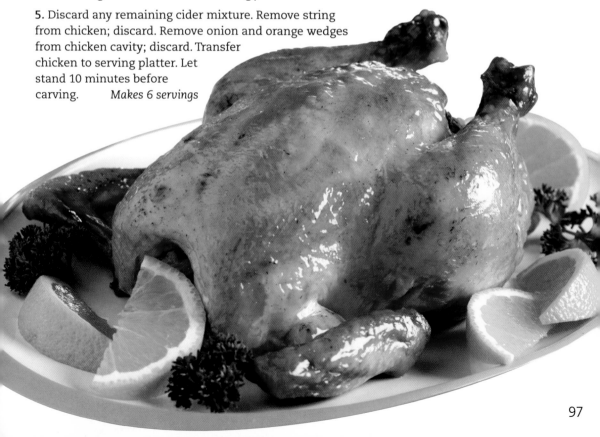

Masa

Masa is the Spanish word for dough. Made from corn that is soaked in lime and then dried, it is gluten-free and traditionally used to make corn tortillas and many other Latin American dishes.

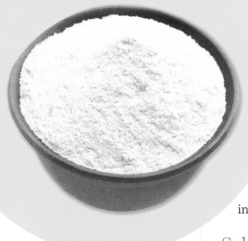

Benefits

Masa can be kind of confusing because it is more of an umbrella term of which there are specific types available that are intended for different uses. When masa is dried it becomes a flour, otherwise known as masa harina, but it is not the same as corn flour or cornmeal. Masa harina is an important ingredient in traditional Mexican cooking, especially because it is used to make ubiquitous corn tortillas and tamales. Instant corn flour is closely related but not the same product, and it is used specifically for making arepas, flat, round corn cakes popular in many Latin American countries. These ingredients are useful for people on a gluten-free diet because they can be used to create a number of foods that can be enjoyed in place of bread or other wheat-containing ingredients.

Selection and Storage

Masa harina can be found near other flours or in the Mexican section of large supermarkets. Instant corn flour for arepas—also called masarepa, masa al instante and harina precodica—is available in Latin American markets and online.

Preparation

For basic, easy-to-make corn tortillas, combine 2 cups masa harina and 1 cup water in a bowl, adding additional water, if necessary, until a ball of dough forms. Break off small sections and flatten to a disc; keep the remaining dough covered to keep moist. Cook the tortillas in an ungreased skillet over medium-high heat 30 seconds, turn over and cook 1 minute, then turn over again and cook 30 seconds or until tortillas are soft, pliable and flecked with brown.

Recipe Suggestions

Use corn tortillas for common Mexican dishes, such as tacos, enchiladas and fajitas, or in place of wheat-containing products in any number of dishes, from sandwiches and wraps to casseroles and even lasagna. Arepas can be topped or filled with a variety of ingredients, including meat, eggs, cheese and veggies. Try making tamales if you are feeling adventurous, and fill them as desired for a delicious, unusual appetizer.

nutrients per serving:

Calories 151	**Carbohydrate** 22g	**Saturated Fat** 3g
Calories from Fat 30%	**Fiber** 4g	**Cholesterol** 11mg
Protein 3g	**Total Fat** 5g	**Sodium** 257mg

arepas (latin american corn cakes)

1½ **cups instant corn flour for arepas***
½ **teaspoon salt**
1½ **to 2 cups hot water**
⅓ **cup shredded Mexican cheese blend**
1 **tablespoon butter, melted**

This corn flour is also called masarepa, masa al instante and harina precodica. It is NOT the same as masa harina or regular cornmeal.

1. Preheat oven to 350°F. Combine instant corn flour for arepas and salt in medium bowl. Stir in 1½ cups water. (Dough should be smooth and moist but not sticky.) Add more water, 1 tablespoonful at a time, if necessary. Add cheese and butter. Knead until dough is consistency of smooth mashed potatoes.

2. Heat heavy skillet or griddle over medium heat. Lightly grease with butter or oil. Break off a piece of dough about the size of an egg; roll into a ball. (If dough cracks or seems too dry, return to bowl and add additional water, 1 tablespoon at a time.)

3. Working in batches, flatten and pat dough into 3- to 4-inch discs, about ½ inch thick. Immediately place in hot skillet. Cook arepas 3 to 5 minutes per side or until browned in spots. Remove to baking sheet.

4. Bake 15 minutes or until arepas sound hollow when tapped.

Makes 6 to 8 arepas
(1 arepa per serving)

Serving Suggestion: To make breakfast sandwiches, split arepas by piercing edges with fork as you would English muffins. Fill with scrambled eggs, cheese and salsa.

Tip: Arepas are best served warm. Day-old arepas are best toasted. Arepas may also be frozen for future use.

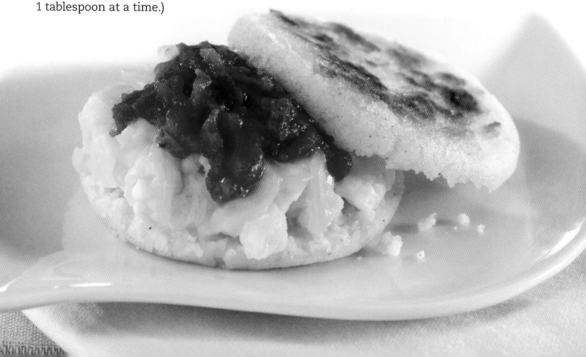

Milk

Cow's milk has been an important part of the human diet for thousands of years and is the most popular animal milk consumed. We enjoy milk—and its cultured relative buttermilk—in countless ways.

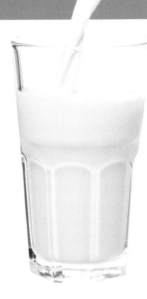

Benefits

Milk is perhaps best known for its role in promoting bone health and preventing osteoporosis, thanks to its high calcium and vitamin D contents. Milk is also rich in high-quality protein. Studies have shown that consuming low-fat milk and milk products can aid weight control, help lower blood pressure and fend off some cancers. Buttermilk shares the same health benefits as milk, with the addition of being a fermented food. Friendly bacteria are added to milk to create buttermilk—thereby making it a probiotic, like yogurt—and the result can help aid digestion and immune function.

Selection and Storage

Milk varies in percentage of fat, from whole (4%) to reduced-fat (2%), low-fat (1%) and fat-free, or skim. Almost all milk sold in the supermarket is homogenized, meaning the fat has been mechanically distributed into the rest of the milk, but some natural food stores carry unhomogenized milk, which you need to shake before consuming in order to incorporate the fat. Some people find the flavor of unhomogenized milk to be richer and truer to traditional milk. Organic milk is frequently available in most supermarkets now. Buttermilk is sold in smaller containers alongside the milk.

Preparation

If you do not have buttermilk for a baking recipe, it's easy to make your own using regular milk. Add enough milk to 1 tablespoon white vinegar or lemon juice in a measuring cup to equal 1 cup; stir and let stand 5 minutes before using. You can also usually substitute buttermilk with plain yogurt.

Recipe Suggestions

Milk is great as part of breakfast, whether on its own, over cold cereal, to make hot cereal or in a fruit smoothie. It is often called for in baking recipes and to make creamy soups, stews and casseroles. Buttermilk can also be enjoyed on its own if you like the rich, tangy flavor, but it is most often used in baking recipes for pancakes, cakes, breads, muffins and biscuits. It also makes a great marinade and tenderizer for chicken and fish.

gluten-free buttermilk pancakes

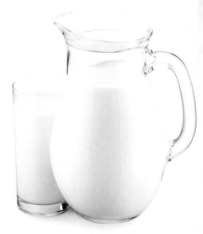

    2 cups Gluten-Free All-Purpose Flour Blend (page 5)*
1½ tablespoons sugar
    1 teaspoon baking powder
    1 teaspoon baking soda
    ½ teaspoon salt
2¼ cups low-fat buttermilk
    2 eggs
    2 tablespoons butter, melted and cooled
       Vegetable oil
       Maple syrup and additional butter

*Or use any all-purpose gluten-free flour blend that does not contain
xanthan gum.

1. Combine flour blend, sugar, baking powder, baking soda and
salt in large bowl. Whisk buttermilk, eggs and 2 tablespoons
butter in small bowl. Gradually whisk buttermilk mixture into
flour mixture until smooth.

2. Heat oil in griddle or large nonstick skillet over medium
heat. Pour ¼ cupfuls batter 2 inches apart onto griddle. Cook
2 minutes or until lightly browned and edges begin to bubble.
Turn over; cook 2 minutes or until lightly browned. Repeat
with remaining batter. Serve with maple syrup and additional
butter.   *Makes 16 pancakes (4 pancakes per serving)*

Note: If you do not plan on serving the pancakes right away,
keep them warm in a 200°F oven until ready to serve.

nutrients per serving:

Calories 409
Calories from Fat 34%
Protein 12g
Carbohydrate 56g
Fiber 2g
Total Fat 16g
Saturated Fat 6g
Cholesterol 114mg
Sodium 960mg

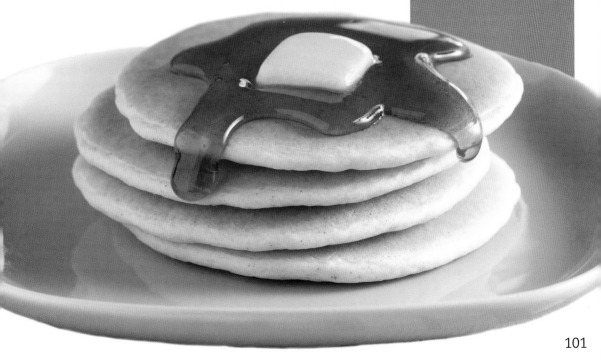

Millet

Millet is one of the earliest cultivated grains, although it's technically a seed. It is most popular in African, Indian and Asian cuisines, and in the United States, it is a common ingredient in birdseed.

Benefits

Like other whole grains, millet is high in protein and fiber and rich in powerful phytonutrients. It is also a good source of the important minerals magnesium and phosphorous. Millet is appreciated as an alternative to some of the more common grains in a gluten-free diet, like rice or even quinoa, and its versatility makes it a great addition to many different kinds of dishes.

Selection and Storage

Millet can be found in packages in large supermarkets or natural food stores along with other grains, and sometimes it is available in bulk bins. Millet looks similar to quinoa in that it has a tiny beaded shape and is a beige color. Store it in a sealed container in a cool, dry, dark place.

Preparation

Rinse and sort though millet before preparing it. Cook millet as you would rice, but use a little more water. The ratio is about 1 cup millet to $2\frac{1}{2}$ to 3 cups water, and you can always use broth instead of water to give it more taste.

It cooks in about 30 minutes and should be tender with slight resistance. To add more flavor to millet, you can toast it for a few minutes in the saucepan before you add the liquid. Millet takes well to different types of seasonings, so use your favorites to boost the interest of the dish by adding them with the millet as it cooks or after it's done.

Recipe Suggestions

Enjoy millet for breakfast as a hot cereal. Try cooking it in part water and part milk, and serve with fruit, nuts and your sweetener of choice. Use millet as an alternate stuffing ingredient for filling vegetables such as eggplant, zucchini, bell peppers or tomatoes. Toss cooked millet with chopped cooked vegetables and meat for a satisfying main dish. It is also excellent on its own as a side dish simply tossed with olive oil and fresh herbs. You can even pop it like popcorn on the stovetop for a crunchy and unique snack.

millet pilaf

- 1 tablespoon olive oil
- ½ onion, finely chopped
- ½ red bell pepper, finely chopped
- 1 carrot, finely chopped
- 2 cloves garlic, minced
- 1 cup uncooked millet
- 3 cups water
- Grated peel and juice of 1 lemon
- ¾ teaspoon salt
- ¼ teaspoon black pepper
- 2 tablespoons chopped fresh parsley (optional)

nutrients per serving:

Calories 164
Calories from Fat 21%
Protein 4g
Carbohydrate 28g
Fiber 4g
Total Fat 4g
Saturated Fat <1g
Cholesterol 0mg
Sodium 304mg

1. Heat oil in medium saucepan over medium heat. Add onion, bell pepper, carrot and garlic; cook and stir 5 minutes or until softened. Add millet; cook and stir 5 minutes or until lightly toasted.

2. Stir in water, lemon peel, lemon juice, salt and black pepper; bring to a boil. Reduce heat to low; cover and simmer 30 minutes or until water is absorbed and millet is tender. Cover and let stand 5 minutes. Fluff with fork. Sprinkle with parsley, if desired.   *Makes 6 servings*

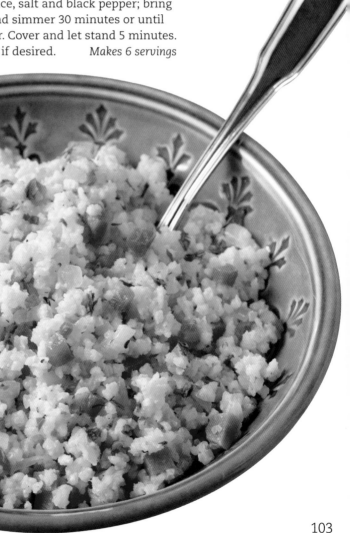

Millet Flour

Millet flour has a mild flavor that verges on slightly nutty and sweet. It is a great addition to gluten-free flour bread blends, particularly for yeast breads, and provides the bread with a texture that is closer to wheat bread.

Benefits

Millet flour retains the health benefits of whole millet, so it is a welcome addition to gluten-free flour bread blends that often contain less nutritionally dense flours and starches. It is easily digested and helps improve the overall nutrition of the bread it produces, particularly by adding fiber, protein and some minerals. It helps create breads that have a light texture and pleasant crust. In addition, it improves the flavor of the bread by contributing its own subtle sweet flavor rather than either the more intense, often beany taste from some gluten-free flours or the bland, weak taste from the starches.

Selection and Storage

Millet flour can be found among specialty flours in natural food stores, usually near other gluten-free foods. Store it in the refrigerator or freezer, where it will stay fresh for several months. Millet flour is more prone to rancidity than some other gluten-free flours, so make sure to store it correctly and don't use it if it smells unusual.

Preparation

Millet flour should generally not be used on its own as the only flour in a recipe. Use it as part of a blend in recipes for yeast breads, including sandwich bread, pizza crust and flat breads. If you like to use gluten-free flour blends, you will find it is an ingredient in many blend recipes, as it is in the flour blend for breads from this book. Millet flour can also be used in combination with other gluten-free flours in baked goods such as pancakes, muffins, cookies and cakes.

Recipe Suggestions

Try substituting part of the brown rice flour called for with millet flour. For most recipes, if you are making something that calls for millet flour but don't have any on hand, you can substitute chickpea flour, but keep in mind that substitution may slightly alter the flavor.

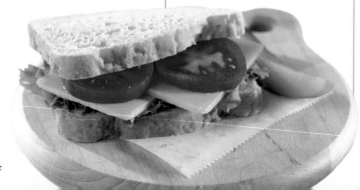

gluten-free pizza

- 1¾ cups Gluten-Free Flour Blend for Breads (page 5)
- 1½ cups white rice flour, plus additional for work surface
- 2 teaspoons sugar
- 1 package (¼ ounce) active dry yeast
- 1½ teaspoons salt
- 1½ teaspoons Italian seasoning
- 1 teaspoon baking powder
- ½ teaspoon xanthan gum
- 1¼ cups hot water (110°F)
- 2 tablespoons olive oil
- Toppings: gluten-free pizza sauce, fresh mozzarella cheese, sliced tomatoes, chopped fresh basil, grated Parmesan cheese

1. Combine flour blend, 1½ cups rice flour, sugar, yeast, salt, Italian seasoning, baking powder and xanthan gum in large bowl. Gradually beat in water with electric mixer at low speed until soft dough ball forms. Add oil; beat 2 minutes.

2. Transfer dough to floured surface and knead 2 minutes or until dough forms smooth ball.

3. Place dough in large greased bowl; turn to coat dough evenly. Cover; let rise in warm place 30 minutes. (Dough will increase in size but not double.)

4. Preheat oven to 400°F. Line pizza pan or baking sheet with foil. Punch down dough and transfer to center of prepared pan. Spread dough as thin as possible (about ⅛ inch thick) using dampened hands.

5. Bake 5 to 7 minutes or until crust just begins to brown. (Crust may crack in spots.)

6. Top crust with desired toppings. Bake 10 to 15 minutes or until cheese is melted and pizza is cooked through.

Makes 4 to 6 servings

nutrients per serving:

Calories 487
Calories from Fat 16%
Protein 7g
Carbohydrate 94g
Fiber 4g
Total Fat 9g
Saturated Fat 1g
Cholesterol 0mg
Sodium 1000mg

Molasses

Molasses used to be the most common sweetener until white sugar became affordable in the early 20th century. Now it's best known for giving gingerbread and baked beans their distinct flavor and dark color.

Benefits

When sugar cane is refined, the resulting juice is boiled down to a syrupy mixture; sugar crystals are then extracted and the remaining liquid is molasses. The first boiling yields light molasses, which is the sweetest, the second yields dark molasses—less sweet—and the third yields blackstrap molasses. Blackstrap molasses is the darkest, thickest and most bitter, but it is also the highest in nutrients. It is an excellent source of iron, calcium and many minerals. All molasses is a healthier choice over refined sweeteners, though, because it has not been stripped of its nutrients. Some find molasses to have too rich of a flavor, but others enjoy it for its complex, bittersweet taste and the way it complements certain baked goods.

Selection and Storage

Generally, light and dark molasses are interchangeable, so many recipes do not specify one or the other. Because blackstrap is so strong, it is usually called for in the ingredient list; do not substitute light for blackstrap or vice versa since the flavor is so different. Molasses is often labeled sulphured or unsulphured, and while it won't make a difference which one you use in a recipe, the unsulphured types generally have a lighter and cleaner taste. Look for light or dark molasses in the baking aisle of supermarkets; blackstrap molasses may be sold there but you can certainly find it at natural food stores. Store molasses tightly covered at room temperature for up to a year.

Preparation

The expression "slow as molasses" is completely true—molasses is so thick that is pours very slowly. When measuring molasses, spray your measuring cup with nonstick cooking spray before adding the molasses to help it slide out with ease.

Recipe Suggestions

Molasses is mostly used in baking recipes, such as for cookies, cakes and gingerbread. Use light molasses when you don't want too powerful of a flavor in recipes or alone as pancake syrup. Dark molasses is best in gingerbread and shoofly pie. Use blackstrap when called for or in savory recipes like baked beans or pulled pork.

gluten-free gingerbread

2 cups Gluten-Free All-Purpose Flour Blend (page 5)*
2 teaspoons ground ginger
¾ teaspoon xanthan gum
½ teaspoon baking powder
½ teaspoon baking soda
½ teaspoon salt
½ teaspoon ground cinnamon
1 cup ginger ale
¾ cup packed brown sugar
6 tablespoons butter, melted and cooled
½ cup molasses
2 eggs
1 tablespoon grated fresh ginger
Whipped cream (optional)

Or use any all-purpose gluten-free flour blend that does not contain xanthan gum.

1. Preheat oven to 350°F. Spray 9-inch square baking pan with nonstick cooking spray.

2. Combine flour blend, ground ginger, xanthan gum, baking powder, baking soda, salt and cinnamon in medium bowl. Whisk ginger ale, brown sugar, butter, molasses, eggs and grated ginger in large bowl until well blended. Add flour mixture in two additions, stirring until well blended after each addition. Pour into prepared pan.

3. Bake 30 to 35 minutes or until toothpick inserted into center comes out clean. Cool in pan 10 minutes. Remove to wire rack to cool slightly. Serve warm or at room temperature with whipped cream, if desired.   *Makes 9 servings*

Tip: For best taste and texture, grate fresh ginger with a microplane zester or with the smallest holes on a box grater.

nutrients per serving:

Calories 328	**Total Fat** 12g
Calories from Fat 31%	**Saturated Fat** 5g
Protein 3g	**Cholesterol** 62mg
Carbohydrate 54g	**Sodium** 324mg
Fiber 1g	

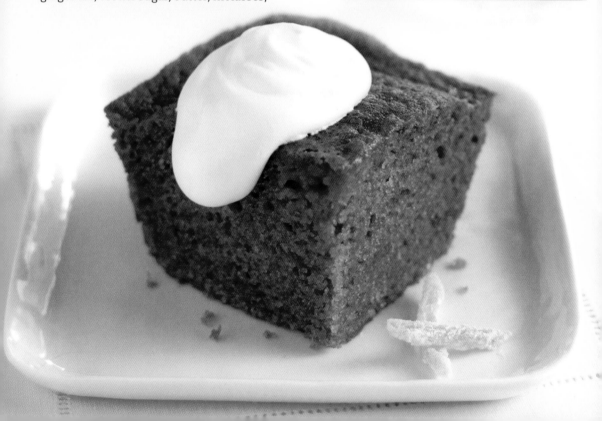

Oats

Oats are a nutritious whole grain and have a place in almost all diets, but they are not without controversy in the gluten-free diet. The bottom line is that oats labeled "gluten-free" are safe for most people with celiac disease.

Benefits

Oats are well known for their hefty amount of soluble fiber, thanks to their bran and germ layers that do not get stripped away during processing. Soluble fiber helps decrease the risk of heart disease and diabetes by lowering blood cholesterol levels and helping to keep blood sugar levels even. Most people who follow a gluten-free diet can reap the benefits of oats, but the main problem is that most oats are processed in facilities that also handle wheat products. Therefore, it is imperative to purchase oats that are certified gluten-free to avoid any cross-contamination with wheat. There does seem to be a small number of people with celiac disease who still have a problem with a particular protein in oats, regardless of the processing. Consult with your doctor for more information and whether you should abstain from any oat products.

Selection and Storage

If you are a celiac patient, you might be limited to the gluten-free oats that are available, which are expensive and not widely available. Look for them at natural food stores or order them online. For others on a less strict gluten-free diet, many types of oats are available. Steel-cut oats are whole oat groats that have been cut into thick pieces. They are heartier, chewier and denser than rolled oats. Rolled oats are oat groats that have been steamed and flattened, and they can be either old-fashioned or quick-cooking, both which are interchangeable. Instant oats are precooked, so they just need to be reconstituted in boiling water, and are not interchangeable with other oats.

Preparation

Cook oats in simmering water or milk until softened. The different kinds of oats require different cooking times, so just follow package directions.

Recipe Suggestions

Oats are most commonly made into oatmeal for a hot breakfast cereal. Dress oatmeal up with fruit and nuts for a well-rounded morning meal. Or make oats into granola for a crunchy snack or addition to yogurt. Oats are also a great addition to cookies and muffins, adding nutrients and chewiness.

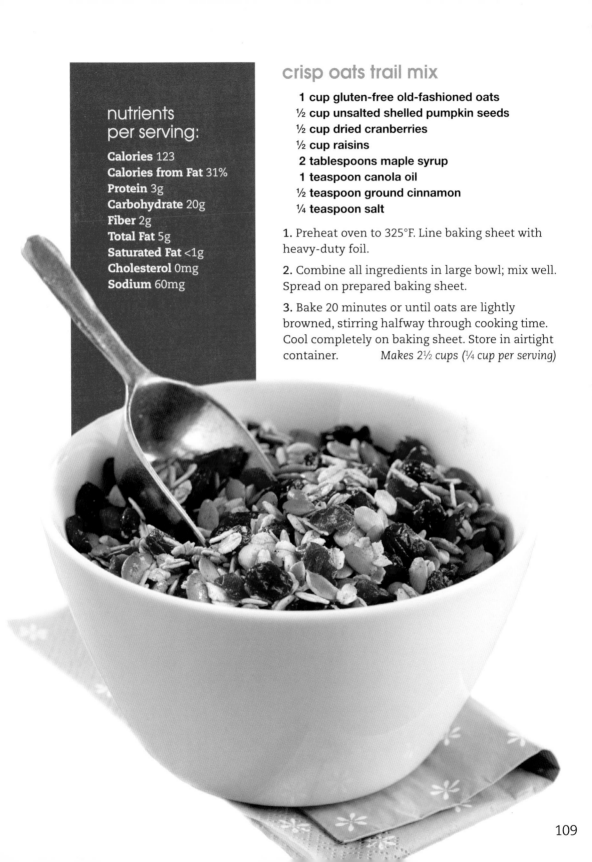

crisp oats trail mix

- **1 cup gluten-free old-fashioned oats**
- **½ cup unsalted shelled pumpkin seeds**
- **½ cup dried cranberries**
- **½ cup raisins**
- **2 tablespoons maple syrup**
- **1 teaspoon canola oil**
- **½ teaspoon ground cinnamon**
- **¼ teaspoon salt**

1. Preheat oven to 325°F. Line baking sheet with heavy-duty foil.

2. Combine all ingredients in large bowl; mix well. Spread on prepared baking sheet.

3. Bake 20 minutes or until oats are lightly browned, stirring halfway through cooking time. Cool completely on baking sheet. Store in airtight container.   *Makes 2½ cups (¼ cup per serving)*

Oat Flour

Oat flour is a fine gluten-free flour alternative as long you can safely consume oat products. Use it for breads and other baked goods as well as to thicken sauces or soups.

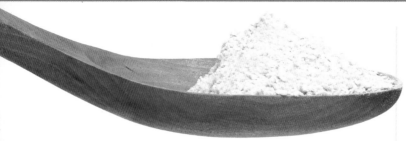

Benefits

Oat flour is made from grinding whole oats into a fine powder. Therefore, it is just as healthful and fiber-rich as oats are. It offers a hefty dose of nutrients in addition to soluble fiber to gluten-free baked goods that are often created using less nutrient-dense flours and starches. It also lends a subtle oaty flavor and blends well with other grain flours for an interesting mix of flavors and textures, creating truly multigrain baked products.

Selection and Storage

As with oats, make sure you buy oat flour that is made from pure oats and is labeled that it is certified gluten-free to avoid any cross-contamination with wheat products. You should be able to find it in natural food stores or you can order it online. Because oat flour contains the nutritious bran and germ of oats, it is prone to rancidity. Store it in the refrigerator or freezer to preserve the quality and flavor.

Preparation

Oat flour is easy to make at home because most people already have oats on hand. Place certified gluten-free old-fashioned oats in the food processor; pulse a few times and then let it run for a minute or until a fine powder is reached. You will need to measure the oat flour after it has been ground to know exactly how much you have. Remember that you will yield less flour than oats that you started with, depending on how you originally measured it, how fine you ground it and how much was lost when transferring it from the food processor.

Recipe Suggestions

Use oat flour with a blend of other gluten-free flours for baking breads, muffins, pancakes, cookies and bars. Try substituting one third of oat flour for another flour if the recipe doesn't already include it. Use oat flour to thicken sauces and soups in place of all-purpose flour, but keep in mind that some chunky soup or chowder recipes call for actual oats, not oat flour.

multigrain sandwich bread

1 cup brown rice flour, plus additional for pan
1 tablespoon active dry yeast (about 1½ packages)
1¾ cups warm water (110°F)
2 tablespoons honey
¾ cup white rice flour
⅔ cup dry milk powder
½ cup gluten-free oat flour
⅓ cup cornstarch
⅓ cup potato starch
¼ cup teff flour
2 teaspoons xanthan gum
2 teaspoons egg white powder
1½ teaspoons salt
1 teaspoon unflavored gelatin
2 eggs
¼ cup canola oil

1. Preheat oven to 350°F. Grease 10×5-inch loaf pan; dust with brown rice flour.

2. Sprinkle yeast over water in medium bowl. Add honey. Cover with plastic wrap; let stand 10 minutes or until foamy.

3. Combine 1 cup brown rice flour, white rice flour, milk powder, oat flour, cornstarch, potato starch, teff flour, xanthan gum, egg white powder, salt and gelatin in large bowl. Stir until well blended.

4. Whisk eggs and oil in small bowl. Gradually beat yeast mixture and egg mixture into flour mixture with electric mixer at low speed until combined. Beat at high speed 5 minutes or until smooth. Pour into prepared pan.

5. Bake 1 hour or until internal temperature reaches 200°F. Remove from pan; cool completely on wire rack.

Makes 12 servings

nutrients per serving:

Calories 272	**Total Fat** 10g
Calories from Fat 32%	**Saturated Fat** 1g
Protein 8g	**Cholesterol** 33mg
Carbohydrate 38g	**Sodium** 348mg
Fiber 2g	

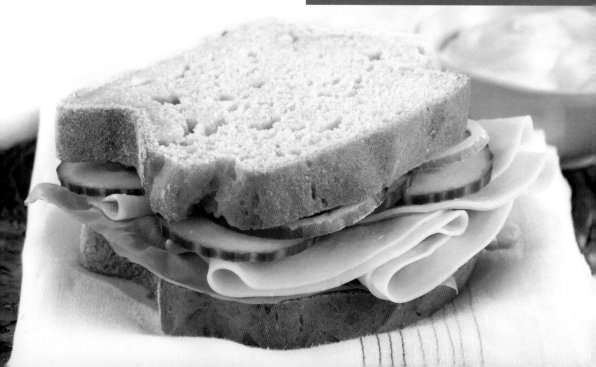

Oranges

This popular citrus fruit offers a sweet, juicy treat with many health benefits. Oranges make wonderful snacks on their own and provide a burst of flavor in recipes.

Benefits

Oranges are abundant in vitamin C. Just one orange provides over 100 percent of the daily requirement for vitamin C. This antioxidant helps protect the heart, ward off infections, heal wounds and maintain healthy teeth and gums. Oranges are also rich in potassium for healthy blood pressure and folate to prevent certain birth defects. They contain some fiber, too, but it's important to eat the whole fruit (as opposed to drinking orange juice) in order to get the full benefits.

Selection and Storage

The most common varieties of oranges for snacking are seedless navels and Valencias, which are also the most common oranges for juicing. Blood oranges—the smaller, aromatic, red-fleshed orange—are less common but are also great to eat on their own. Mandarin oranges are loose skinned, easily sectioned and can be sweet or tart; they are also available canned. Oranges are available year-round but are at their peak in the winter months, usually when you most need a fresh, juicy treat. Select firm fruit that are heavy for their size, which indicates they are juiciest. Store them in the refrigerator up to a couple weeks. Choose orange juice not from concentrate and with no added sugars.

Preparation

Oranges come encased in a protective skin, so only peeling is necessary in order to enjoy them. Choose seedless oranges for snacking and use in fruit salads. If a recipe calls for a small amount of orange juice, you can squeeze your own for the best flavor. Roll a room-temperature orange on the counter under your palm, cut the fruit in half and squeeze into a measuring cup. For orange zest, wash the orange well and use a microplane grater, if possible, to get a very fine grate and avoid the bitter white pith.

Recipe Suggestions

Oranges make great snacks on their own or additions to fruit salads, green salads and yogurt parfaits. Orange juice can be a great ingredient in marinades, dressings and sauces for meats and other main dishes. And don't forget about the endless ways of creating smoothies using orange juice, yogurt and any combination of fruit.

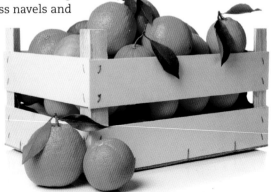

Peanut Butter

This beloved American food is only about a century old, but it's hard to imagine not having it in most of our diets. This protein-rich treat is wonderful no matter how you spread it.

Benefits

Made from ground peanuts, peanut butter shares most of its health benefits with the whole nut. Peanut butter is high in fat, but the majority of it is monounsaturated, so it helps lower bad cholesterol and improve good cholesterol, thereby having a positive influence on overall heart health. Also rich in protein and fiber, peanut butter digests slowly and keeps you satisfied for longer. Peanuts offer the benefits of many vitamins and minerals as well, including vitamin E, niacin and iron. Peanut butter is most often a favorite for sandwiches, but its uses go beyond the humble lunch or snack and can be incorporated into many baked goods and even main dishes.

Selection and Storage

Most commercial peanut butters contain oil, sugar and salt in addition to peanuts, and these varieties are preferred for the convenience of being shelf stable and not having to stir. However, the traditional or natural style has a richer peanut flavor and texture and is better for you because it only contains peanuts and sometimes salt. It does need to be stirred when it is first opened and then refrigerated. Look for natural peanut butter in glass jars along with the other peanut butters in the supermarket. Some large grocery stores offer machines that grind peanuts right there so you get the freshest product possible.

Preparation

It's easy to make your own peanut butter, and you can't beat the freshness and superior flavor. Just process shelled peanuts in the food processor for a few minutes, scraping down the side occasionally, until the desired consistency is reached. Add a small amount of oil (peanut or olive) or even water or milk to add creaminess. Use unsalted nuts so you can add salt to taste. Keep covered in the refrigerator or freezer.

Recipe Suggestions

Use peanut butter as a spread on toast, crackers, apples, bananas or celery. Add it to baked goods like cookies, bars and quick breads. It even can be a delicious addition to many Asian-style dishes in the form of a rich, sweet and salty peanut sauce.

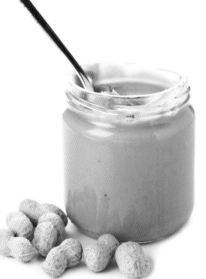

Pecans

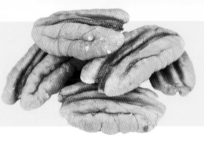

This popular tree nut is native to North America and is still cultivated in the southern states, which is one of the reasons they play an important role in Southern cuisine.

Benefits

Pecans are nutrient dense and pack a healthy punch in a small portion. They are rich in disease-fighting antioxidants, particularly vitamin E, which helps protect the heart. They are a good source of potassium, calcium and magnesium, all which help promote healthy blood pressure. They also contain protein and fiber to keep you full. What's more, pecans help reduce bad cholesterol levels while increasing good cholesterol thanks to their plant sterols. Pecans are loved not only for their health benefits but also for their rich, buttery taste and versatility in recipes. Great on their own as a snack, they can also be added to many sweet and savory dishes for added crunch and flavor.

Selection and Storage

Pecans naturally come in a hard, thin shell, but you will almost always find them unshelled. They may be sold in bulk bins or in packages of halves, chips or ground nuts. They are also available raw or roasted and salted or unsalted. Choose unsalted raw pecans for using in recipes, but you may prefer to snack on the salted roasted variety. Store shelled pecans tightly sealed in a cool, dry place for three months, in the refrigerator for nine months or in the freezer for two years.

Preparation

Raw pecans benefit from being toasted before adding them to recipes. Spread them in a single layer on a

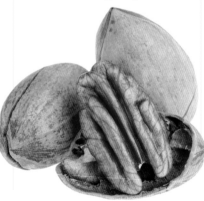

baking sheet and bake in a 350°F oven for 5 to 7 minutes or until lightly browned and fragrant, stirring occasionally. To create your own ground pecans, grind pecan halves in the food processor by pulsing until coarse crumbs form, but be careful not to overprocess and create pecan butter.

Recipe Suggestions

Use toasted pecan halves to top salads and vegetable dishes. Add pecan chips to cereal or yogurt. Pecans make a wonderful addition to many baked goods, such as cookies, cakes, muffins, quick breads and pancakes. They are commonly added to many Southern sweets, including famous pecan pie, carrot cake and even the frosting for red velvet cake. Ground pecans make a wonderful high-protein, crunchy coating for chicken or fish in place of bread crumbs.

pecan catfish with cranberry compote

Cranberry Compote (recipe follows)
2 tablespoons butter, divided
1½ cups pecans
2 tablespoons rice flour
1 egg
2 tablespoons water
Salt and black pepper
4 catfish fillets (about 1¼ pounds)

1. Preheat oven to 425°F. Prepare Cranberry Compote; set aside.

2. Melt 1 tablespoon butter; place in 13×9-inch baking pan, tilting pan to distribute evenly.

3. Combine pecans and rice flour in food processor; pulse just until finely chopped.

4. Place pecan mixture in shallow dish. Whisk egg and water in another shallow dish. Sprinkle salt and pepper on both sides of each fillet. Dip fillets in egg mixture, then in pecan mixture, pressing to adhere. Place fillets in prepared pan in single layer. Dot with remaining 1 tablespoon butter.

5. Bake 15 to 20 minutes or until fish begins to flake when tested with fork. Serve with Cranberry Compote.　　*Makes 4 servings*

cranberry compote

1 package (12 ounces) fresh cranberries
¾ cup water
⅔ cup sugar
¼ cup orange juice
2 teaspoons grated fresh ginger
¼ teaspoon Chinese five-spice powder
⅛ teaspoon salt
1 teaspoon butter

1. Wash and pick over cranberries, discarding any bad ones. Combine cranberries and all remaining ingredients except butter in large saucepan. Cook over medium-high heat 10 minutes or until berries begin to pop, stirring occasionally.

2. Cook and stir 5 minutes or until sauce is thickened. Remove from heat; stir in butter until melted. Let stand 10 minutes.

Makes about 3 cups

Note: Compote can be made up to one week ahead and stored in the refrigerator.

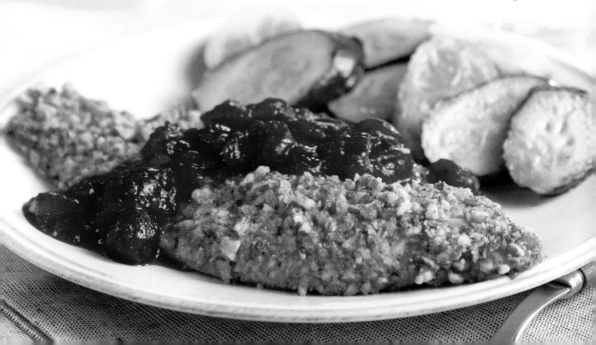

Pectin

Pectin, a complex carbohydrate naturally found in many fruits, particularly the peels of citrus fruits, may be best known as an ingredient in jams and jellies, but it is also suitable for use in gluten-free baking.

Benefits

Pectin is important for making jams and jellies because it properly thickens without adding any flavor. Pectin's primary function as an ingredient in gluten-free baking is as a thickener and binder, which is important in recipes where there is not enough jelling action present. Gelatin also serves this purpose, but for those who follow a vegan diet, pectin is an excellent substitute. In addition to helping bind ingredients, it helps retain moisture in the final product, both important functions when baking gluten-free bread. Pectin is also added as a stabilizer to some commercial foods such as certain dairy products and baked goods. Beyond its cooking applications, pectin is available as a dietary supplement in capsule form as a source of fiber to help improve digestion.

Selection and Storage

Pectin is available in liquid and dry, powdered form, although the powder is more common. Either can be used for making jams or jellies, but you will want to use the powder for gluten-free breads. Pectin can be found in the specialty baking section of large supermarkets or natural food stores. It is available in pouches inside small boxes. It keeps indefinitely when stored in a cool, dry place.

Preparation

In addition to being useful for jams and jellies, pectin is an excellent thickener for other jelled foods, such as aspic, pie filling and even yogurt. Some pectin requires a particular level of sugar to be present in order to work, but there are other varieties available that are geared towards low-sugar recipes. Just follow the recipe directions in order to properly dissolve the pectin, and be aware that the food does not completely jell until it cools.

Recipe Suggestions

For gluten-free breads, if there is gelatin in the recipe already, just substitute it with the same amount of pectin. You can also try and add 1 teaspoon of pectin to a bread recipe even if gelatin is not called for. Unlike gelatin, pectin does not need to be dissolved because it is simply combined with the other dry ingredients.

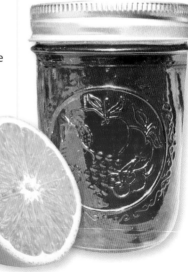

asiago garlic rolls

1 cup warm water (110°F)
1 package (¼ ounce) active dry yeast
1 teaspoon sugar
3 eggs
¼ cup extra virgin olive oil
½ teaspoon cider vinegar
1½ cups Gluten-Free Flour Blend for Breads
  (page 5)
½ cup cornstarch
¼ cup almond flour
1¼ teaspoons xanthan gum
1 teaspoon powdered pectin or unflavored
  gelatin
½ teaspoon salt
½ cup plus 2 tablespoons grated Asiago
  cheese, divided
6 cloves roasted garlic*
1 tablespoon chopped fresh rosemary
  leaves

*To roast garlic, preheat oven to 375°F. Remove outer
layers of papery skin and cut off top of garlic head.
Place cut side up on a piece of heavy-duty foil. Drizzle
with 2 teaspoons olive oil; wrap in foil. Bake 25 to
30 minutes or until cloves feel soft when pressed.
Cool slightly before squeezing out garlic pulp.

1. Grease 12 standard (2½-inch) muffin cups. Combine water, yeast and sugar in small bowl; let stand 10 minutes or until foamy.

2. Whisk eggs, oil and vinegar in medium bowl. Combine flour blend, cornstarch, almond flour, xanthan gum, pectin and salt in large bowl. Beat in yeast mixture and egg mixture with electric mixer at low speed. Stir in ½ cup cheese, garlic and rosemary. Beat at high speed 3 minutes or until smooth.

3. Spoon batter into prepared muffin cups, filling three-fourths full. Cover with plastic wrap sprayed with nonstick cooking spray. Let rise in warm place 30 minutes.

4. Preheat oven to 375°F.

5. Bake 15 minutes. Sprinkle rolls with remaining 2 tablespoons cheese. Bake 5 to 10 minutes or until lightly browned. Remove to wire rack; cool completely.

Makes 12 rolls

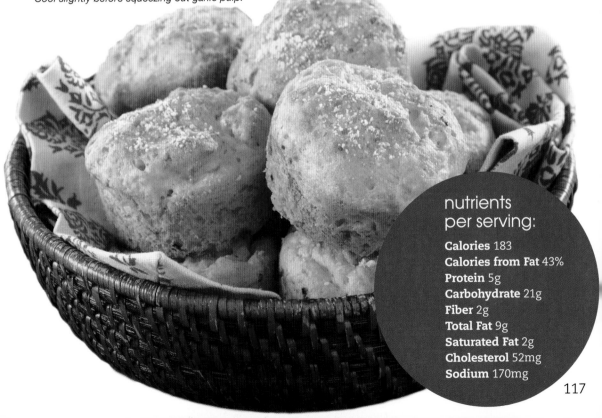

nutrients per serving:

Calories 183
Calories from Fat 43%
Protein 5g
Carbohydrate 21g
Fiber 2g
Total Fat 9g
Saturated Fat 2g
Cholesterol 52mg
Sodium 170mg

117

Plantains

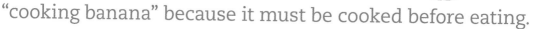

This fruit might be mistaken for a large banana—it is in fact a type of banana—but it is actually quite different. It's referred to as a "cooking banana" because it must be cooked before eating.

Benefits

Plantains are quite starchy and full of carbohydrates. They are a good source of potassium, magnesium, fiber and vitamin C. Even though they are a fruit, they are often considered to be a vegetable due to their common uses. They range in ripeness and can be used at any stage, but it does affect their texture and flavor. Unripe green plantains are the starchiest, whereas ripe brown-speckled or even black-skin plantains are the sweetest. Popular in Latin American countries and the Caribbean, they are a unique food to learn how to prepare and introduce into your diet.

Selection and Storage

Plantains are sold in the produce section of most supermarkets. If selection is slim or nonexistent there, look for them in Mexican grocery stores. They look like very large bananas. Select firm, unripe ones that you can then ripen at home. Store them at room temperature and turn daily; it will take about a week for them to ripen.

Preparation

Plantains have to be cooked in order to eat them; what makes them so great is that this can be done in many ways. Unripe plantains are commonly made into plantain chips, or tostones. Heat a large skillet of oil to 350°F. To peel the tough skin of green plantains, slice off the ends of plantains, slit the skin lengthwise with a sharp knife, then remove the skin. Cut into 1-inch slices and fry for 3 minutes. Drain on paper towels and then flatten into thin discs. Fry them again for 3 minutes or until crisp. Drain on paper towels and season with salt. Or to cook sweet plantains, slice very ripe plantains into ½-inch slices; brush with oil, season with salt and bake on a baking sheet in a 450°F oven for 15 minutes or until very tender.

Recipe Suggestions

Enjoy plantain chips as a snack or appetizer on their own or with a dip like guacamole. Or serve them as an accompaniment to any soup, stew or casserole. Softer baked or sautéed plantains go very well with rice and beans as a side dish. You can even wrap them in corn tortillas and top with cheese and salsa for unusual but delicious vegetarian enchiladas.

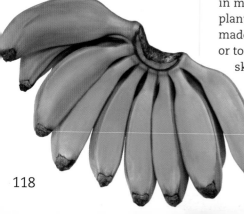

exotic veggie chips

3 tropical tubers (malanga, yautia, lila and/or taro roots)*

1 to 2 green (unripe) plantains

2 parsnips, peeled

1 medium sweet potato, peeled

1 lotus root**

Vegetable oil for deep frying

Coarse salt

*These tropical tubers are all similar and their labels are frequently interchangeable or overlapping. They are available in the produce section of Latin markets. Choose whichever tubers are available and fresh. Look for firm roots without signs of mildew or soft spots.

**Lotus root is available in the produce section of Asian markets. The outside looks like a fat beige link sausage, but when sliced, the lacy, snowflake-like pattern inside is revealed.

1. Line baking sheets with paper towels. Fill deep fryer or large heavy skillet with oil; heat to 350°F on deep-fry thermometer.

2. Peel thick shaggy skin from tubers, rinse and dry. Slice tubers and place in single layer on prepared baking sheets to absorb excess moisture. (Stack in multiple layers with paper towels between layers.) Peel thick skin from plantain. Slice and arrange on paper towels.

Slice parsnips and sweet potato and arrange on paper towels. Trim lotus root and remove tough skin with paring knife. Slice and arrange on paper towels.

3. Working in batches, deep fry each vegetable until crisp and slightly curled, stirring occasionally. (Frying time will vary from 2 to 6 minutes depending on the vegetable.)

4. Remove vegetables with slotted spoon and drain on paper towels; immediately sprinkle with salt. Cool completely. Store in airtight containers at room temperature. *Makes about 6 servings*

Note: To recrisp chips, bake in preheated 350°F oven 5 minutes.

nutrients per serving:

Calories 288	**Total Fat** 6g
Calories from Fat 19%	**Saturated Fat** 1g
Protein 4g	**Cholesterol** 0mg
Carbohydrate 58g	**Sodium** 56mg
Fiber 6g	

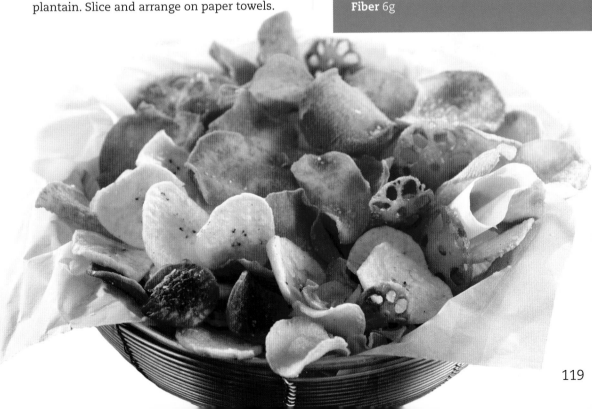

Polenta

Polenta is a staple of Northern Italy and even more commonly eaten there than pasta. This soft, hearty dish is perfect comfort food on its own or dressed up with sauces and other accompaniments.

Benefits

Polenta gives you the same health benefits of corn as long as you make it with whole grain, or stone-ground, cornmeal. Polenta can be made from whole cornmeal or degerminated cornmeal, in which the nutritious germ has been removed. Refined cornmeal might make polenta faster to cook, but the nutrition, texture and flavor of polenta made from whole cornmeal is best. Polenta is a popular alternative to bread and pasta, and it has many uses beyond a basic side dish that are worth exploring.

Selection and Storage

You can make polenta from cornmeal, which comes in white and yellow as well as fine and coarse grinds. You can also make it from corn grits, which are sometimes also labeled "polenta." Thanks to the increasing popularity of polenta, you can now easily find quick-cooking and instant polenta as well as precooked polenta in plastic tubes. Look for these products with other grains and starches in the supermarket. Precooked polenta must be stored in the refrigerator after opening.

Preparation

Preparing polenta from whole cornmeal can be somewhat of a slow, involved process, but it should not be rushed in order to ensure the best and creamiest texture. Bring 4 cups of water to a boil in a saucepan. Slowly stir in 1 cup cornmeal and continue stirring for about 30 minutes. It's important not to stop stirring, and if the water runs low, just add a little bit more. The longer you cook and stir, the creamier the final product will be. To make polenta solid, pour the cooked polenta into a greased baking pan and let cool until firm. Then you can cut it into pieces and bake, broil or grill.

Recipe Suggestions

Polenta is creamy and delicious on its own, but it can always be made into a more substantial dish by adding any kind of cheese, vegetables or meat. Use firm polenta slices in lasagna or top it like pizza. Polenta also makes a great hearty breakfast, either savory topped with a poached egg or sweet topped with fruit and maple syrup.

polenta pizzas

1 teaspoon olive oil
½ cup chopped onion
¼ pound bulk mild Italian sausage
1 can (8 ounces) gluten-free pizza sauce
1 roll (16 ounces) prepared polenta
1 cup (4 ounces) shredded mozzarella cheese

1. Preheat oven to 350°F. Spray 13×9-inch baking pan with nonstick cooking spray.

2. Heat oil in large skillet over medium heat. Add onion; cook and stir 3 minutes or until tender. Add sausage; brown 5 minutes, stirring to break up meat. Stir in pizza sauce; simmer 5 minutes.

3. Cut polenta roll into 16 slices; arrange in prepared pan. Spoon 1 heaping tablespoon sausage mixture over each polenta slice. Sprinkle 1 tablespoon cheese over each slice.

4. Bake 15 minutes or until polenta is hot and cheese is melted.   *Makes 4 servings (4 pizzas per serving)*

nutrients per serving:

Calories 322
Calories from Fat 40%
Protein 15g
Carbohydrate 32g
Fiber 2g
Total Fat 14g
Saturated Fat 7g
Cholesterol 36mg
Sodium 968mg

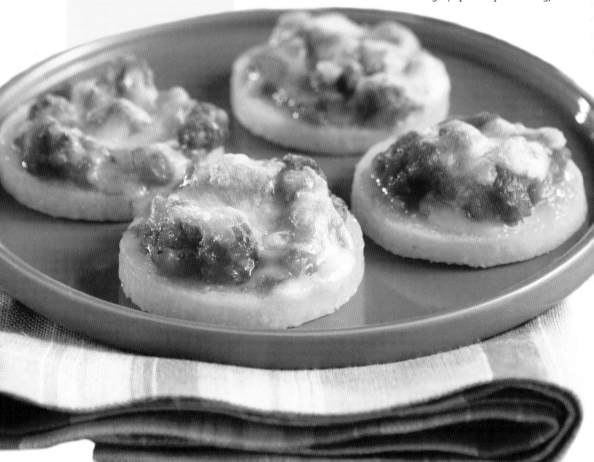

Popcorn

Everyone's favorite snack at the movies is also a great snack for people on a gluten-free diet. Because corn is naturally gluten-free, popcorn is as well.

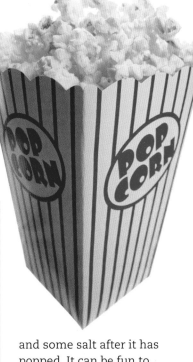

Benefits

Popcorn is considered a whole grain because it is made from corn. It contains a decent amount of fiber, very few calories and no fat. However, this is assuming that the popcorn has been air-popped and eaten plain. Most people prefer popcorn oil-popped and topped with butter or other flavorings. Keep in mind that while you still get the benefits of corn when eating flavored popcorn, you also are getting the less desirable calories, fat, sodium and sometimes sugar from the additives.

Selection and Storage

Popcorn is available at the supermarket in microwavable packages in a wide array of flavors. You can also find it at gourmet popcorn stores in some cities and to order online. Keep in mind that while much of the commercial popcorn available is gluten-free, you should always check labels thoroughly to be safe. Some brands may add gluten-containing ingredients or manufacture their popcorn with other gluten-containing foods. Although it's not nearly as common anymore, you can always buy old-fashioned kernels ready for popping at home on the stovetop. This way your popcorn is sure to be gluten-free and healthier than prepared options. Popping corn is available in yellow, white and even red and blue varieties. Store it in an airtight container at room temperature for about a year.

Preparation

Follow package directions for preparing popcorn in the microwave or on the stovetop. When making your own popcorn from popping corn, leave it plain or add melted butter and some salt after it has popped. It can be fun to try adding different types of seasonings for variety— try smoked paprika, chili powder, curry powder, ground cumin or grated Parmesan cheese.

Recipe Suggestions

Beyond enjoying popcorn as a simple snack on its own, it can be mixed with a number of other ingredients. For a fun treat, combine plain popcorn with any combination of gluten-free cereals, nuts and dried fruits, toss with melted butter and any desired seasonings (go savory with salt and dried herbs or sweet with sugar or honey), then bake at 350°F for about 15 minutes.

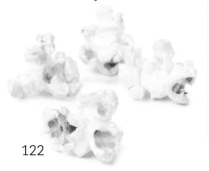

Pork

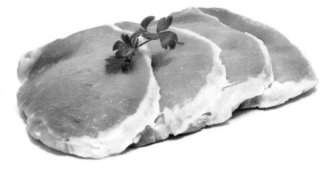

Benefits

Pork is rich in high-quality protein, which helps keep you satisfied, and many B vitamins, including thiamin, niacin, riboflavin and vitamin B_6. These B vitamins are essential to everyone, and they're especially important to get enough of because their natural sources are more limited than those of many other essential nutrients. Pork also supplies a good amount of phosphorous, zinc and potassium. Pork products vary considerably in fat content, with pork tenderloin being the leanest; it is comparable to skinless chicken breast in calories and fat.

Selection and Storage

Most pork is cured, or processed—including bacon, ham and sausage—while the rest is fresh—including pork tenderloin, pork chops, pork loin and ground pork. Be sure to read the labels of processed pork products to ensure they are gluten-free. Most pork products are available raw in the fresh or frozen meat section of the supermarket. You can also find a wide variety of fully cooked pork products (primarily the cured kinds)

Pork is a wonderful alternative to chicken. There are many types of pork available and plenty of ways to cook it. Pork makes a great center of a meal or flavor enhancer for vegetable dishes.

both refrigerated and frozen. Fresh pork should be stored, wrapped well, in the refrigerator for up to three days. It can be frozen, also wrapped well, for up to six months.

Preparation

Fresh pork should be cooked until it has an internal temperature of 145°F; it will appear slightly pink in the center. The USDA recently lowered the temperature from 160°F, so now you can enjoy pork

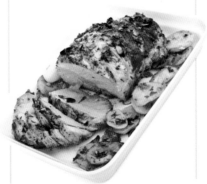

safely while keeping it moist and flavorful. After cooking you should let it rest for a few minutes to let the temperature finish rising and seal the juices in the meat.

Recipe Suggestions

Fresh pork has a mild flavor, so it's best when prepared with a spice rub, marinade or flavorful sauce when served on its own. You can stuff thick pork chops with a number of fillings, such as a fruit and nut mixture, finely chopped vegetables or wild or regular rice. Chop up pork tenderloin for a stir-fry, casserole or pasta dish. Cured pork can stand on its own as a main dish, but thanks to its full flavor, it makes a great addition to soups, stews, egg dishes and vegetables.

123

Potatoes

America's favorite vegetable is also one of the ideal comfort foods. Potatoes are an important food staple around the world and are economical, versatile and surprisingly nutritious.

Benefits

Potatoes are a very healthful food as long as they're not prepared in the beloved manner of fries and chips or loaded down with unhealthy ingredients. They are a good source of immune-boosting vitamin C, blood pressure-lowering potassium and filling fiber. It is important to eat the skin along with the flesh to take advantage of all the available nutrients.

Selection and Storage

There are hundreds of varieties of potatoes, although most of us are familiar with just a few. Russets, also known as

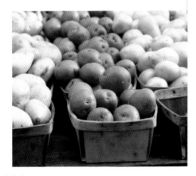

baking potatoes, are perhaps the most common. Due to their starchy, fluffy interior, they are best suited to baking or mashing. Waxy potatoes—including round red and round white—have less starch and more moisture and are better used for boiling, roasting or grilling. New potatoes are simply young potatoes and have a waxy texture and thin skins. Fingerling potatoes are cute and little and available at farmers' markets in a wide array of colors, including gold, red, blue and purple. Choose firm potatoes free of green spots or sprouts. Store them in a dry, cool, dark place away from onions; do not refrigerate them. Mature potatoes will last for several weeks, but new potatoes only last a few days to a week.

Preparation

Scrub potatoes well and cut off any sprouts or bad spots before cooking. Bake pierced whole potatoes in the oven at 350°F for about an hour or in the microwave for about 10 minutes. For healthier French fries, thinly slice potatoes and toss with olive oil, salt and pepper on a baking sheet; roast at 400°F for about 30 minutes.

Recipe Suggestions

Top baked potatoes with plain Greek yogurt, shredded cheese and sliced green onions. Mash cooked potatoes with olive oil, roasted garlic, salt and pepper. Toss potatoes with other root vegetables, like carrots, parsnips and onions, add olive oil and dried herbs and roast together for a hearty and healthy side dish. Or create a Niçoise salad with new potatoes, tomatoes, green beans, black olives, onions, tuna and hard-cooked eggs, tossed in an herbed vinaigrette.

bacon, potato and cheddar anytime frittata

4 slices turkey bacon
2 teaspoons olive oil, divided
½ cup finely chopped green bell pepper
½ cup finely chopped red bell pepper
½ cup finely chopped onion
1 cup frozen shredded potatoes or hash brown potatoes, partially thawed
2 eggs, lightly beaten
¼ teaspoon salt
⅛ teaspoon black pepper
⅛ teaspoon dried thyme
2 tablespoons finely shredded reduced-fat Cheddar cheese

1. Heat small nonstick skillet over medium-high heat. Add bacon; cook 3 minutes or until browned. Remove to plate. When cool enough to handle, cut bacon into small pieces.

2. Heat 1 teaspoon oil in same skillet. Add bell peppers and onion; cook and stir 3 to 4 minutes or until onion is translucent.

3. Reduce heat to medium-low. Sprinkle potatoes over vegetables in skillet. Drizzle remaining 1 teaspoon oil evenly over potatoes. Carefully pour in eggs; sprinkle evenly with salt, black pepper and thyme. Top evenly with bacon. Cover and cook 10 minutes or until knife inserted near center comes out clean.

4. Remove from heat; sprinkle evenly with cheese. Cover and let stand 2 minutes or until cheese is melted. To serve, cut into wedges.

Makes 2 servings
(2 wedges per serving)

nutrients per serving:

Calories 321
Calories from Fat 48%
Protein 17g
Carbohydrate 25g
Fiber 3g
Total Fat 17g
Saturated Fat 5g
Cholesterol 213mg
Sodium 969mg

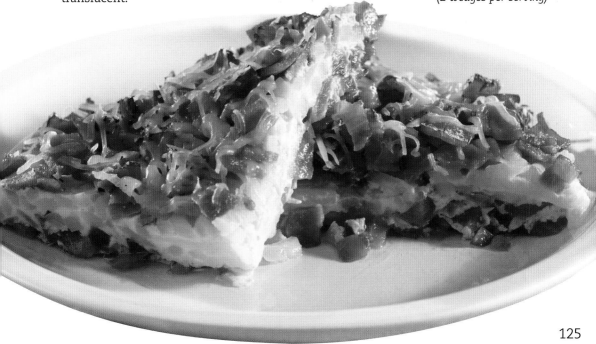

Potato Flakes

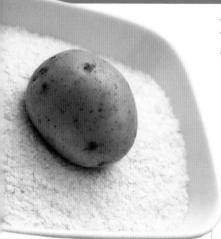

Potato flakes may be most familiar to you as instant mashed potatoes. These flakes of dried potatoes can do more than just make a quick and easy side dish; they are a useful addition to a gluten-free pantry.

Benefits

Potato flakes are not as nutritious as whole potatoes because they are a processed product of them, but they do retain a small amount of fiber, protein and vitamin C. It is generally best to get health benefits from a complete food, so potato flakes should be used more as a supporting ingredient instead of the main star of a meal. Potato flakes are a good addition to gluten-free breads, giving them more moisture and body, and they also make an excellent coating for chicken or fish instead of bread crumbs.

Selection and Storage

Instant potato flakes are widely available in boxes or pouches in the supermarket.

Plain, unflavored potato flakes should only be used in gluten-free baking recipes. There are also a number of different flavors available, but those are primarily intended for use as a side dish on their own and may not be gluten-free.

Preparation

To make mashed potatoes from potato flakes, the flakes need to be reconstituted in water and milk. Simply follow the package directions to do so. For use in gluten-free

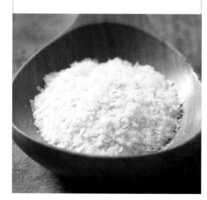

baking, potato flakes can either be part of a gluten-free flour blend (as they are in the blend for breads in this book) or added to a baking recipe that uses a blend without potato flakes.

Recipe Suggestions

If not using a flour blend that already includes potato flakes, try adding up to ¼ cup with the other dry ingredients. Or use potato flakes for more than just baking. Try a mixture of potato flakes and Parmesan cheese as a coating for chicken or fish. Dip the meat first into potato flour mixed with desired seasonings, then into a beaten egg, then into the potato flakes before baking or sautéing. Potato flakes can also be used in place of bread crumbs in meatballs or seafood patties.

olive & herb focaccia

- 3 cups Gluten-Free Flour Blend for Breads (page 5)
- 2 packages (¼ ounce each) active dry yeast
- 2 teaspoons xanthan gum
- 1 teaspoon salt
- 1¼ cups warm water (110°F), divided
- ¼ cup extra virgin olive oil
- 3 egg whites
- 1 tablespoon honey
- 1 teaspoon cider vinegar

Toppings

- 1 cup chopped pitted kalamata olives
- 3 tablespoons chopped fresh rosemary leaves
- 2 tablespoons chopped fresh thyme
- 3 cloves garlic, minced
- ¼ cup extra virgin olive oil
- Salt and black pepper
- ¼ cup grated Romano cheese

1. Combine flour blend, yeast, xanthan gum and 1 teaspoon salt in large bowl. Whisk 1 cup water, ¼ cup oil, egg whites, honey and vinegar in medium bowl until well blended. Beat into dry ingredients with electric mixer at low speed until combined. (Batter should be smooth, shiny and thick.) Add more water, 1 tablespoon at a time, if necessary. Beat at medium-high speed 5 minutes, scraping bowl occasionally.

2. Preheat oven to 450°F. Line pizza pan or baking sheet with parchment paper or foil. Place dough in center of prepared pan. Using wet hands, spread dough into two 8-inch rounds, about ½ inch thick. Let rest 20 minutes.

3. Dimple tops of dough rounds with fingertips or back of wooden spoon. Sprinkle evenly with olives, rosemary, thyme and garlic. Drizzle with ¼ cup oil. Sprinkle with salt and pepper.

4. Bake 15 minutes or until lightly browned. Immediately sprinkle with cheese. Cool slightly on wire rack before slicing.

Makes 2 focaccia breads
(about 24 servings)

nutrients per serving:

Calories 114	**Total Fat** 6g
Calories from Fat 45%	**Saturated Fat** 1g
Protein 2g	**Cholesterol** 1mg
Carbohydrate 14g	**Sodium** 157mg
Fiber 1g	

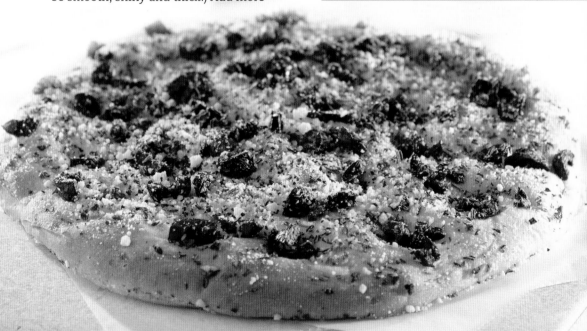

Potato Starch

Be careful not to confuse potato starch with potato flour. Potato starch is produced from only the starch of potatoes, whereas potato flour is produced from the whole potato.

Benefits

Potato starch is a good ingredient to use for thickening liquids such as gravies, sauces, soups and stews, and it is an excellent substitute for all-purpose flour in these instances. In gluten-free baking, potato starch helps yield light and moist baked goods. Potato starch is similar in appearance and function to cornstarch, tapioca starch and arrowroot. Although they have subtle differences, they are close enough that they are suitable substitutes for one another, and their bland tastes will not noticeably alter the flavor of the dish. For commercial uses, potato starch is added to some processed foods such as instant soup as a thickener and even grated cheese to prevent clumps.

Selection and Storage

Potato starch is most often found among specialty flours in large supermarkets or natural food stores, usually near other gluten-free foods. Make sure not to accidentally buy potato flour. The starch is lighter and whiter than the flour and closely resembles cornstarch. Store it in the refrigerator or freezer, where it will stay fresh for several months.

Preparation

When using potato starch as a thickener, be sure to mix it with a liquid before adding it to the dish to properly dissolve it and avoid lumps. It will thicken quickly once you add it. For gluten-free baking, potato starch is frequently called for both in various baking mixes and in flour blends, either instead of or in addition to another starch, depending on the blend and its intended use.

Recipe Suggestions

Use potato starch in a gluten-free flour blend for muffins, quick breads and yeast breads for a moist and tender texture. Of course, there are prepared blends available to purchase as well as many different recipes for blends, but you might want to try experimenting making your own, as there are numerous variations possible. This way you can play with substituting starches (as well as the different flours) and see what kind of results they yield.

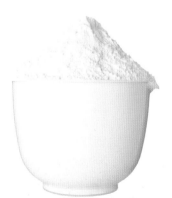

vegetable-bean chowder

- 1 tablespoon olive oil
- ½ cup chopped onion
- ½ cup chopped celery
- 3 cups water
- 1½ teaspoons salt
- 2 cups cubed peeled potatoes
- 1 cup sliced carrots
- 1 can (15 ounces) cream-style corn
- 1 can (about 15 ounces) cannellini or navy beans, rinsed and drained
- ¼ teaspoon dried tarragon
- ¼ teaspoon black pepper
- 2 cups whole milk
- 1 tablespoon potato starch

1. Heat oil in large saucepan or Dutch oven over medium heat. Add onion and celery; cook and stir 3 minutes or until crisp-tender. Add water and salt. Bring to a boil over high heat. Add potatoes and carrots. Reduce heat to medium; cover and simmer 10 minutes or until potatoes and carrots are tender.

2. Stir in corn, beans, tarragon and pepper. Cover and simmer 10 minutes or until heated through.

3. Stir milk into potato starch in medium bowl until smooth. Stir into vegetable mixture. Simmer, uncovered, until thickened. *Makes 5 servings*

nutrients per serving:

Calories 297
Calories from Fat 20%
Protein 11g
Carbohydrate 51g
Fiber 7g
Total Fat 7g
Saturated Fat 2g
Cholesterol 10mg
Sodium 1211mg

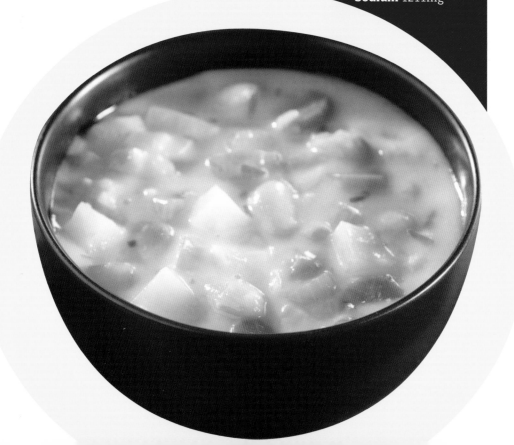

Pumpkin

Pumpkin goes well beyond jack-o'-lanterns and Thanksgiving pie. Pumpkin and its seeds (also known as pepitas) can be enjoyed in many ways, from sweet to savory and from a snack to a main dish.

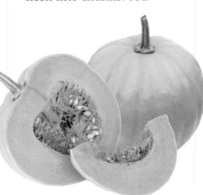

Benefits

The bright orange color of pumpkin is an indicator that it is rich in antioxidant beta-carotene (vitamin A), which helps prevent certain cancers. Pumpkin is also a good source of vitamin C, iron, potassium and fiber. Pumpkin seeds are rich in protein and a good source of iron and healthy unsaturated fat.

Selection and Storage

The best pumpkins for eating are not the same ones used for jack-o'-lanterns; they are smaller and called pie or sugar pumpkins. Pumpkins are available in the fall and winter and keep well for a month in a cool, dry place. Canned pumpkin is available and a convenient choice if you just need a puree. Pumpkin pie filling is also available, but due to its added sugar and spices, it is not a substitute for regular pumpkin.

Preparation

To prepare pumpkin purée from a whole pumpkin, cut it in half and remove the pulp and seeds. Bake the pumpkin halves on a baking sheet at 350°F for 45 minutes or until the flesh is tender. Scrape out the flesh with a spoon and mash it. If you want pumpkin pieces, peel a whole pumpkin, cut it in half, remove the pulp and seeds, then cut the flesh into chunks. You can then roast, bake, boil or microwave the pieces. Don't discard the pumpkin seeds; separate them from the stringy pulp, rinse and dry them, then bake on a greased baking sheet at 350°F for 20 minutes. Lightly salt them or add other seasonings.

Recipe Suggestions

Pumpkin purée can be made into soups, stews, cookies, quick breads or pies. Add it to casseroles or make it into a rich sauce for pasta dishes. Use cooked chunks as a side dish or mix it with other roasted autumn vegetables to serve with quinoa or rice. Pumpkin can be substituted for butternut squash or even sweet potato in some recipes. Enjoy pumpkin seeds as a crunchy snack with other seeds and nuts or in trail mix. They can be sprinkled on soups and salads or baked into muffins and cookies.

gluten-free pumpkin muffins

2¼ cups Gluten-Free All-Purpose Flour Blend (page 5)*
½ teaspoon salt
½ teaspoon ground ginger
½ teaspoon ground nutmeg
½ teaspoon xanthan gum
¼ teaspoon baking soda
1 cup packed dark brown sugar
1 cup canned pumpkin
½ cup (1 stick) butter, melted and cooled
¼ cup low-fat buttermilk
2 eggs
3 tablespoons molasses
1 teaspoon vanilla

Or use any all-purpose gluten-free flour blend that does not contain xanthan gum.

1. Preheat oven to 400°F. Spray 12 standard (2½-inch) muffin cups with nonstick cooking spray.

2. Combine flour blend, salt, ginger, nutmeg, xanthan gum and baking soda in medium bowl. Whisk brown sugar, pumpkin, butter, buttermilk, eggs, molasses and vanilla in large bowl. Add flour mixture in two additions, stirring until well blended after each addition. Spoon evenly into prepared muffin cups.**

3. Bake 18 to 22 minutes or until toothpick inserted into centers comes out clean. Cool in pan 5 minutes. Remove to wire rack to cool slightly. Serve warm or at room temperature.

Makes 12 muffins

**For best results, scoop batter into each muffin cup in a single scoop, filling to the top, and do not add additional batter.*

Note: Do not substitute pumpkin pie mix for the canned pumpkin. It produces an overly sweet and spiced muffin.

nutrients per serving:

Calories 268
Calories from Fat 36%
Protein 3g
Carbohydrate 41g
Fiber 2g
Total Fat 11g
Saturated Fat 5g
Cholesterol 52mg
Sodium 217mg

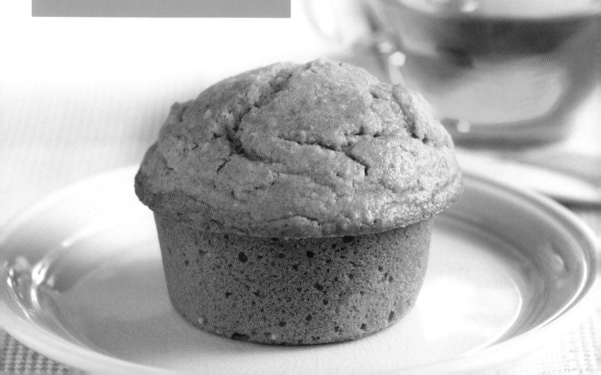

Quinoa

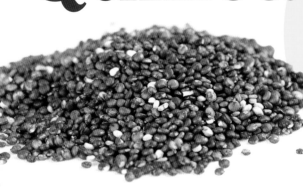

Although it is just recently gaining popularity in the United States, quinoa has been cultivated in South America for thousands of years and remains a staple there. It has been referred to by the Incas as the "mother seed."

Benefits

Quinoa is often referred to as a superfood because it is so healthful. It stands out among the whole grains because it has more protein than any other grain and is lower in carbohydrates, too. It is a good source of fiber, calcium, iron and other important minerals, too. Quinoa is a good substitute for other grains you might be tired of, such as rice. It is also a good stand-in for couscous and bulgur wheat, which are not permitted in a gluten-free diet.

Selection and Storage

Quinoa can be found in packages in large supermarkets or natural food stores along with other grains, and sometimes it is available in bulk bins. Quinoa has a tiny beaded shape and is most commonly ivory colored, although it is also available as red and black. Store it in a sealed container in a cool, dark, dry place.

Preparation

Some people like to rinse quinoa in a fine-mesh strainer before cooking. The seeds are naturally coated with a substance called saponin, which imparts a bitter taste. It is usually rinsed during processing, so you might not notice any off flavor, but it is something to be aware of if you are sensitive to

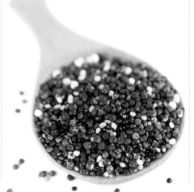

bitterness. Cook quinoa like rice, using one part quinoa to two parts water or broth. It cooks in 15 minutes and will expand to four times its size and become light and translucent. Because quinoa is so versatile, you can accentuate it with any of your favorite seasonings.

Recipe Suggestions

Quinoa has so many serving possibilities, so feel free to use it as you would any other grain, including as a side dish on its own or as a stuffing for a variety of vegetables. Add it to soups, salads and main dishes to bulk up the dish with nutrients, interesting texture and a subtle, nutty flavor. You can even make it with milk as a hot cereal and add fruit, nuts, cinnamon and any desired sweetener.

wild mushroom quinoa stuffing

- 1 cup uncooked quinoa
- 2 tablespoons olive oil, divided
- 2 cups gluten-free vegetable broth
- 1 teaspoon poultry seasoning
- ½ teaspoon salt
- 1 small onion, diced
- 8 ounces cremini mushrooms, sliced
- 8 ounces shiitake mushrooms, stemmed and sliced
- ½ cup diced celery
- 2 tablespoons chopped fresh parsley (optional)

1. Place quinoa in fine-mesh strainer; rinse well under cold running water.

2. Heat 1 tablespoon oil in medium saucepan over medium-high heat. Add quinoa; stir until evenly coated. Stir in broth, poultry seasoning and salt. Bring to a boil. Reduce heat to low; cover and simmer 15 to 20 minutes or until liquid is absorbed. Remove from heat.

3. Meanwhile, heat remaining 1 tablespoon oil in large skillet over medium heat. Add onion, mushrooms and celery; cook and stir 8 to 10 minutes or until vegetables are tender.

4. Combine quinoa and vegetables in large bowl. Sprinkle with parsley, if desired.   *Makes 6 servings*

nutrients per serving:

Calories 181
Calories from Fat 31%
Protein 7g
Carbohydrate 25g
Fiber 4g
Total Fat 6g
Saturated Fat 1g
Cholesterol 0mg
Sodium 392mg

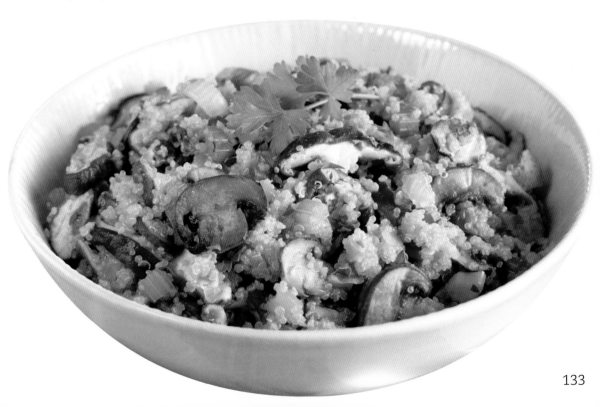

133

Quinoa Flour

If you enjoy cooking and eating whole quinoa, you will love it ground into flour. Quinoa flour maintains the superb healthful properties of quinoa as well as its delightful nutty flavor.

Benefits

One of the primary advantages of using quinoa flour as opposed to other gluten-free flours is that it's superiorly healthful. Quinoa flour stands out against other gluten-free flours and starches due to its vital nutrients, including high protein and fiber contents, as well as its easy digestibility. It makes a good addition to gluten-free flour blends because it helps mask the less appetizing tastes of the bean flours with its pleasantly nutty flavor. It also helps lighten baked goods that would otherwise be weighed down by the heavier bean flours. Quinoa flour, oftentimes along with corn flour, is also made into gluten-free pasta, which is a welcome sight for anyone who misses traditional gluten-containing pasta.

Selection and Storage

Quinoa flour is most often found among specialty flours in natural food stores, usually near other gluten-free foods. Different brands vary in taste and texture, so try different ones to find the one you like best. Store it in the refrigerator or freezer, where it will stay fresh for several months.

Preparation

Although not very common in prepared gluten-free flour blends, quinoa flour is easy to add to baked goods such as cookies, cakes, muffins, pancakes and breads. It pairs especially well with almond flour, buckwheat flour, chickpea flour and soy flour.

Recipe Suggestions

Experiment with replacing some of the gluten-free flour called for in a recipe with quinoa flour. You might find that replacing half is a good starting point to get a feel for how it affects the final dish without completely altering it. There is a possibility of using all quinoa flour for a baked good, but it is best to find a recipe that has been successfully tested using all quinoa flour. Take advantage of the variety of pastas made with quinoa flour, and use them in any recipe that calls for regular pasta.

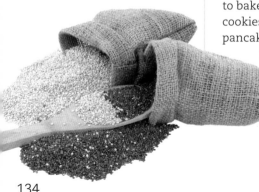

raspberry clafouti

3 eggs*
⅓ cup sugar
1 cup half-and-half
2 tablespoons butter, melted and
    slightly cooled
½ teaspoon vanilla
⅓ cup quinoa flour
⅓ cup almond flour
    Pinch salt
2 containers (6 ounces each) fresh
    raspberries

Use the highest quality eggs possible since the flavor of this dessert depends upon them.

1. Preheat oven to 325°F. Generously butter 9-inch ceramic tart pan or pie plate.

2. Beat eggs and sugar in large bowl with electric mixer at medium speed 4 minutes or until slightly thickened. Add half-and-half, butter and vanilla; whisk to combine. Gradually whisk in quinoa flour, almond flour and salt.

Pour enough batter into prepared pan to just cover bottom. Bake 10 minutes or until set.

3. Remove from oven. Scatter raspberries evenly over baked batter. Stir remaining batter and pour over raspberries.

4. Bake 40 to 45 minutes or until center is set and top is golden. Cool completely on wire rack. Refrigerate leftovers.   *Makes 8 to 10 servings*

nutrients per serving:

Calories 190
Calories from Fat 53%
Protein 5g
Carbohydrate 19g
Fiber 4g
Total Fat 11g
Saturated Fat 5g
Cholesterol 90mg
Sodium 45mg

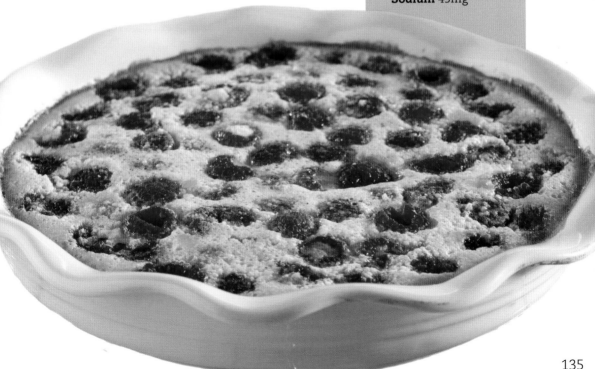

Raisins

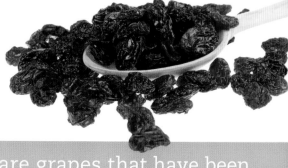

Benefits

Raisins are rich in phenols, which are antioxidants found in fruit that help prevent damage to the body's cells. Raisins contain fewer phenols than fresh grapes, but they are still a good source of them, particularly antioxidant flavonols. Raisins are also a good source of fiber, iron and some minerals. They are very high in natural sugars, however, so they should be eaten in moderation.

Selection and Storage

There are many varieties of raisins, but the most common snacking kind are dark colored and seedless. Golden raisins are made from grapes that have been treated to prevent their color from darkening and dried mechanically, so the result is a more moist and plump raisin. Currants are similar to raisins but are made from Zante grapes and are smaller and primarily used in baking. Raisins come in bulk and a variety of packages, with the small boxes being a good choice to take with you as an easy, gluten-free snack. Raisins should be stored at room temperature for up to about six months.

Raisins are grapes that have been dried by the sun naturally or in the oven mechanically. They make a great snack and are a welcome addition to many types of dishes, especially baked goods.

Preparation

Raisins can always just be eaten straight from the package, which is why they make such a great snack. You may want to soak them (alone or mixed with other dried fruits) in a small bowl of warm water to soften them for use in hot dishes like fruit compote. Add them to baked goods for a burst of moistness and sweetness.

Recipe Suggestions

Enjoy raisins as a snack on their own or in trail mix with gluten-free cereal, other dried fruits, nuts and chocolate chips. Bake them into cookies, cakes, breads and muffins. Add them to baked fruit desserts like apple crisp. Sprinkle them on cereal or yogurt for breakfast. They can go savory, too, like mixed into chicken or tuna salad or sprinkled on a green salad. Or add them to a rice dish, stuffing or a vegetable such as spinach. Serve a golden raisin compote with chicken or duck for an elegant entrée.

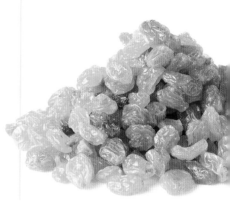

gluten-free fruit cake

2 cups Gluten-Free All-Purpose Flour Blend
    (page 5),* plus additional for pan
1½ teaspoons xanthan gum
1 teaspoon baking powder
1 teaspoon grated fresh ginger
1 teaspoon ground cinnamon
½ teaspoon baking soda
½ teaspoon salt
½ teaspoon ground cloves
2 cups packed dark brown sugar
1 cup (2 sticks) butter, softened
6 eggs
½ cup orange juice
¼ cup molasses
2 cups golden raisins
1½ cups chopped dried apricots
1 cup chopped walnuts
1 cup chopped pecans
1 cup dried cranberries
    Powdered sugar (optional)

Or use any all-purpose gluten-free flour blend that does not contain xanthan gum.

1. Preheat oven to 300°F. Spray 10-inch bundt pan with nonstick cooking spray; dust with flour blend.

2. Combine 2 cups flour blend, xanthan gum, baking powder, ginger, cinnamon, baking soda, salt and cloves in large bowl. Beat brown sugar and butter in medium bowl with electric mixer at medium-high speed 3 minutes or until light and fluffy.

3. Add eggs, one at a time, beating at medium speed until well blended after each addition. Add orange juice and molasses; beat at low speed until well blended. Gradually add flour mixture; beat at medium speed 2 minutes. Fold in raisins, apricots, walnuts, pecans and cranberries. Pour into prepared pan.

4. Bake 2 to 2½ hours or until toothpick inserted near center comes out clean.** Cool in pan on wire rack 1 hour. Remove to wire rack; cool completely. Sprinkle with powdered sugar, if desired.

Makes 12 servings

**If cake becomes too dark on top, tent loosely with foil for last 30 to 60 minutes of baking time.*

Note: You can use any combination of your favorite dried fruits and nuts in this recipe.

nutrients per serving:

Calories 701	**Total Fat** 33g
Calories from Fat 41%	**Saturated Fat** 12g
Protein 9g	**Cholesterol** 134mg
Carbohydrate 101g	**Sodium** 247mg
Fiber 6g	

Rice

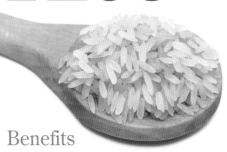

This ancient grain is perhaps the most important grain for people who can't eat gluten. Beyond the thousands of varieties of rice, it can be made into numerous products that are very useful in a gluten-free diet.

Benefits

Brown rice (a whole grain) is the healthier choice over white rice. Brown rice includes the nutritious bran and germ that are stripped away when rice is milled and polished to create white rice. Brown rice is rich in protein, fiber, minerals manganese, selenium and magnesium, and some of the B vitamins. White rice retains a little protein and fiber but loses the bulk of them plus much of the essential minerals and vitamins found in brown rice.

Selection and Storage

Rice is categorized by its size: long grain, medium grain or short grain. Long grain rice produces grains that are dry and separate easily. Short grain rice, like arborio rice, produces grains with the highest starch content, which causes them to be moist and stick together. Medium grain rice is between the two. Popular varieties include Arborio (used for risotto), basmati (aromatic and nutty), jasmine (soft textured and aromatic) and sweet rice (used for sushi). Rice is widely available in supermarkets, and you may be able to find less common kinds in ethnic markets or natural food stores, including red or black varieties. Rice should be stored at room temperature, but brown rice has a shorter shelf life than white, about six months.

Preparation

Cook rice in a saucepan on the stovetop with twice as much liquid (water or broth) as dry grains. Follow package directions for cooking time, but it is more or less done when all the liquid is absorbed. To flavor rice before cooking, sauté finely chopped vegetables and dried herbs or spices in olive oil, then add the rice and toast it for a few minutes. When aromatic and golden, add the liquid, cover and cook for the appropriate time.

Recipe Suggestions

Serve rice as a side dish, plain with butter, salt and pepper or with desired flavorings. Top it with any kind of cooked meat and vegetables for a complete meal. Bake it into casseroles or add it to soups and stews. Make a cold salad using rice and an assortment of chopped fresh veggies and herbs.

Rice Cakes

Rice cakes are a great gluten-free snack and can even be a suitable substitute for bread in a sandwich. Crunchy and light, enjoy them plain, flavored or with your favorite toppings.

Benefits

Plain rice cakes are made just of rice and salt. Usually the rice is brown, so they contain a small amount of protein and fiber and count as a whole grain. Because the rice is puffed, they are light and airy and have few calories. They have a subtle flavor, so they make an excellent snack any time of the day. Used in place of bread in a sandwich, they contribute a satisfyingly crunchy texture to your midday meal. The plain variety of rice cake is rather bland and therefore suited to any type of topping or filling.

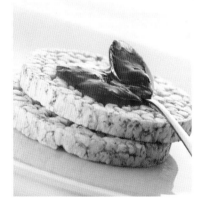

Selection and Storage

Rice cakes come plain and in different flavors, both savory and sweet. They come in standard size or minis, which are also called rice snacks. They can be found with other snack foods or crackers in the supermarket. Rice cakes did not all used to be gluten-free, but since there has been an increased demand for gluten-free products, most large rice cake manufacturers started producing gluten-free rice cakes and labeling them as such. Check the label if you're unsure to be safe. Rice cakes should be kept sealed at room temperature to prevent them from going stale.

Preparation

Rice cakes are prepared and packaged, so they require no work whatsoever. Enjoying them is as simple as eating them straight out of the package or else spreading or topping them as desired.

Recipe Suggestions

Spread plain rice cakes with peanut butter and top with sliced apple or banana, or fill two rice cakes with sliced deli meat and fresh veggies for a snack or light lunch. Make sweet flavors of rice cakes into dessert by topping them with whipped cream, sliced fresh fruit and ice cream topping. Break plain or savory flavors of rice cakes into bite-size pieces and mix them with any gluten-free cereal for a party mix. Combine the mixture with some melted butter and seasoning of your choice (try chili powder or Italian seasoning), then bake at 300°F for 15 minutes. Store in a well-sealed container to maintain freshness.

Rice Crackers

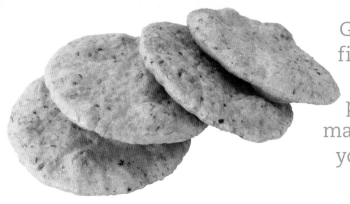

Get your crunchy snack fix with gluten-free rice crackers. They can be purchased packaged in many different flavors, but you can also easily make your own from scratch.

Benefits

Rice crackers are a welcome treat for anyone on a gluten-free diet since they can be substituted for any kind of wheat-containing cracker in any recipe. Rice crackers made with brown rice have better nutrition than those made with white rice, as brown rice contains more protein and fiber.

Selection and Storage

Rice crackers can also be called rice thins or rice crisps depending on the brand. They are made from either brown or white rice and come plain as well as in a variety of flavors. As the gluten-free diet gains more recognition, especially as it has in the past few years, many manufacturers are expanding their gluten-free offerings, giving you much more selection among your favorite packaged foods, including crackers, in the supermarket. Look for rice crackers with other crackers or in the gluten-free aisle in large supermarkets. Be aware that many if not all of the rice cracker party mixes, also known as Japanese rice crackers, that contain an assortment of small rice crackers with seasoning do contain gluten because they are made with soy sauce. Make sure the package you purchase states that it is gluten-free.

Preparation

In addition to purchasing many kinds of prepared rice crackers, you can make them at home as well. You can find simple recipes online or in gluten-free cookbooks, including this one to get you started.

Note that they require few ingredients and a short baking time, so you can whip up a batch at almost any time.

Recipe Suggestions

Use rice crackers anywhere you would regular crackers. Eat them alone as a snack or topped with cheese or any kind of dip as an appetizer. Serve them alongside soups and salads or use crushed crackers as a crunchy topping. Try using them crushed and sprinkled over casseroles for a nice crispy crust.

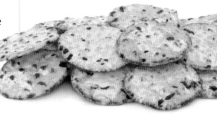

gluten-free cheddar crackers

1½ cups brown rice flour
1 teaspoon garlic powder
1 teaspoon salt-free Italian seasoning
½ teaspoon salt
½ cup (2 ounces) finely grated sharp Cheddar cheese
6 tablespoons cold butter, cut into ½-inch cubes
½ cup water

1. Combine brown rice flour, garlic powder, Italian seasoning and salt in food processor or blender; process until well blended. Add cheese and butter; pulse until evenly incorporated. Add water; process until dough forms.

2. Divide dough into two pieces; wrap in plastic wrap and refrigerate 20 minutes.

3. Preheat oven to 350°F. Line baking sheets with parchment paper.

4. Place each dough half between two pieces of parchment paper; roll out to ⅟₁₆-inch thickness. Refrigerate 3 to 5 minutes.

5. Cut dough into 2½-inch squares; place on prepared baking sheets.

6. Bake 15 minutes or until golden and crisp, rotating after 10 minutes. Cool on baking sheets 10 minutes. Remove to wire racks; cool completely.

Makes 24 crackers (4 crackers per serving)

nutrients per serving:

Calories 283
Calories from Fat 50%
Protein 5g
Carbohydrate 31g
Fiber 2g

Total Fat 16g
Saturated Fat 9g
Cholesterol 40mg
Sodium 358mg

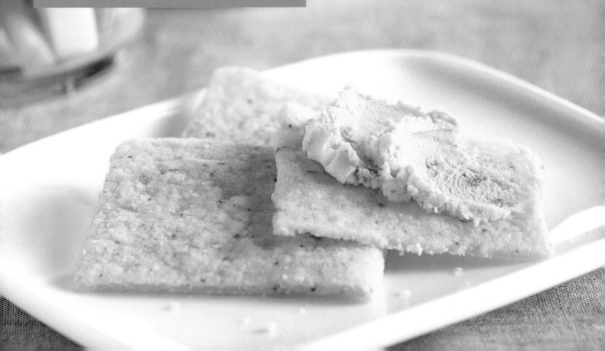

Rice Noodles

These semi-translucent dried noodles are made from rice and are therefore a great go-to ingredient for gluten-free diets, perfect for a variety of Asian dishes or as a substitute for pasta.

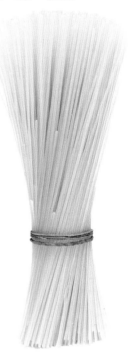

Benefits

Most rice noodles are made only of rice flour and water. They are mostly carbohydrates but do offer a small amount of protein and fiber. Where they really shine is as a substitute for wheat-containing pasta or other noodles in gluten-free diets. Use them in place of regular vermicelli or spaghetti, Chinese wheat or egg noodles, chow mein noodles or bean threads.

Selection and Storage

Rice noodles are sometimes labeled rice-flour noodles, rice sticks or rice vermicelli. They come in a variety of widths, from string thin (usually called rice vermicelli or thin rice sticks) to medium to wide. All rice noodles can be used interchangeably. Make sure to check the ingredient list since occasionally they contain wheat flour

as well. Rice noodles are usually sold dried in bunches and can be found at Asian markets or in the Asian section of large supermarkets. You may be able to find fresh rice noodles refrigerated or frozen in large Asian grocery stores.

Preparation

Rice noodles need to be soaked to soften them before using. Soak them in a large bowl of hot water for 15 to 20 minutes or until soft. Drain and use as directed. You can then boil presoaked rice noodles for a couple minutes, but it's not always necessary. Sometimes just mixing them into a stir-fry or soup for a couple minutes is sufficient in order to reheat them and blend the flavors. Thin rice noodles can also be deep-fried until they puff up and become crunchy. Do not soak them, but instead immerse the dry noodles

into a wok of hot vegetable oil for a few seconds. (You might need to hold them under the oil with tongs.) Quickly remove them and drain on paper towels.

Recipe Suggestions

Add softened rice noodles to any stir-fry or soup. Use them softened at room temperature or deep-fried as a bed for cold salads like Chinese chicken salad. Add softened thin rice noodles to fresh spring rolls or any other wrap that's held together with rice paper wrappers.

basil chicken with rice noodles

1 pound boneless skinless chicken breasts, cut into bite-size pieces
5 tablespoons gluten-free soy sauce, divided
1 tablespoon white wine or rice wine
3 cloves garlic, minced
1 tablespoon grated fresh ginger
8 ounces uncooked rice noodles
  Juice of 2 limes
2 tablespoons packed brown sugar
1 tablespoon vegetable oil
1 red onion, sliced
1 yellow or red bell pepper, cut into strips
2 medium carrots, cut into matchstick-size pieces
2 jalapeño or serrano peppers,* chopped
1½ cups loosely packed basil leaves, shredded

*Jalapeño peppers can sting and irritate the skin, so wear rubber gloves when handling peppers and do not touch your eyes.

1. Place chicken in shallow dish. Combine 3 tablespoons soy sauce, wine, garlic and ginger in small bowl. Pour over chicken and stir to coat. Marinate at room temperature 30 minutes or refrigerate up to 2 hours.

2. Place rice noodles in medium bowl. Cover with hot water; let stand 15 minutes or until tender. Drain.

3. Whisk remaining 2 tablespoons soy sauce, lime juice and brown sugar in small bowl until sugar is dissolved.

4. Heat oil in large skillet or wok over medium-high heat. Add chicken with marinade; cook and stir 5 minutes or until cooked through. Add onion, bell pepper, carrots and jalapeño peppers; cook and stir 4 to 6 minutes or until vegetables are crisp-tender.

5. Stir sauce and add to skillet; cook and stir 2 minutes. Add rice noodles and basil; toss to combine.   *Makes 4 to 6 servings*

nutrients per serving:

Calories 460	**Total Fat** 7g
Calories from Fat 14%	**Saturated Fat** 1g
Protein 29g	**Cholesterol** 72mg
Carbohydrate 69g	**Sodium** 1504mg
Fiber 3g	

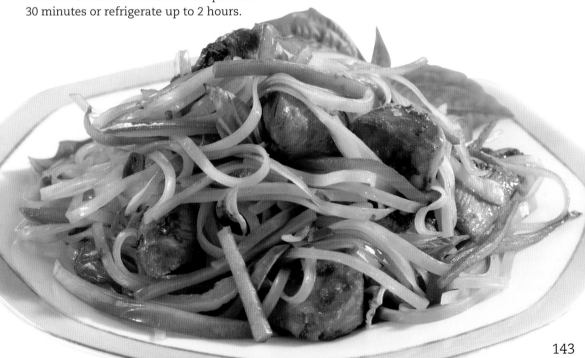

Rice Paper Wrappers

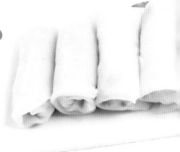

You may know rice paper wrappers as the outside of fresh spring rolls. They are thin, edible wrappers used in Southeast Asian cooking and perfect for a gluten-free diet.

Benefits

Rice paper wrappers are made simply from rice flour, water and salt, sometimes with the addition of tapioca starch. Therefore, they are thin, light and very low in calories. Used primarily for wrapping Vietnamese spring rolls, rice paper wrappers also make a good gluten-free substitute for other wrappers that contain wheat, including egg roll wrappers, wonton wrappers, flour tortillas and even lasagna noodles in some instances.

Selection and Storage

Also known as spring roll wrappers, Vietnamese rice paper or banh trang, rice paper wrappers are a dry product available at Asian markets. They can also be purchased at some other specialty markets or online. They come either round or square and in a variety of sizes. Store them in a cool, dark place for several months.

Preparation

Rice paper wrappers are brittle, so they need to be softened before you use them. Simply soak them in a bowl of warm water for about 30 seconds or until soft and pliable. They will dry out if you don't use them right away, so either work with one or two at a time or else cover the softened wrappers with a damp towel. Rice paper wrappers are most often used fresh, but they can be cooked as well.

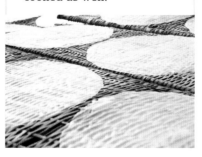

Recipe Suggestions

Use rice paper wrappers to make traditional fresh spring rolls, or fill with any combination of fresh veggies and herbs, cooked seafood or meat and softened rice noodles. You can actually use rice paper wrappers to wrap almost anything, even to make your favorite sandwich into a wrap without the bread. They can be used to wrap any kind of salad, from fresh green salads to tuna or chicken salad. Beyond using them fresh, try filling them as desired and then deep-frying, like for egg rolls. You can even use them for homemade ravioli in place of wonton wrappers or in lasagna in place of lasagna noodles, but keep in mind that due to their thinness and neutral taste, they blend in with the filling much more.

vietnamese summer rolls

Vietnamese Dipping Sauce (recipe follows)
8 ounces medium raw shrimp, peeled and deveined
3½ ounces uncooked thin rice noodles (rice vermicelli)
12 rice paper wrappers, about 6½ inches in diameter
36 whole fresh cilantro leaves
4 ounces roast pork or beef, sliced ⅛ inch thick
1 tablespoon chopped peanuts
Lime peel strips (optional)

1. Prepare Vietnamese Dipping Sauce; set aside.

2. Bring large saucepan of water to a boil over high heat. Add shrimp; simmer 1 to 2 minutes or until shrimp are pink and opaque. Remove with slotted spoon to small bowl. When cool enough to handle, slice in half lengthwise.

3. Meanwhile, place rice noodles in medium bowl. Cover with hot water; let stand 15 minutes or until tender. Drain; cut noodles into 3-inch lengths.

4. Working with one or two at a time, soften rice paper wrappers in large bowl of warm water 30 to 40 seconds or until pliable. Drain on paper towels and transfer to clean work surface. Arrange three cilantro leaves in center of wrapper. Layer with two shrimp halves, pork and rice noodles.

5. Fold bottom of wrapper up over filling; fold in each side and roll up to enclose filling. Repeat with remaining wrappers.

6. Sprinkle with peanuts; garnish with lime peel. Serve with Vietnamese Dipping Sauce.

Makes 12 rolls (2 rolls per serving)

vietnamese dipping sauce

½ cup water
¼ cup gluten-free fish sauce
2 tablespoons lime juice
1 tablespoon sugar
1 clove garlic, minced
¼ teaspoon chili oil

Combine all ingredients in small bowl; mix well. *Makes about 1 cup*

nutrients per serving:

Calories 236
Calories from Fat 12%
Protein 15g
Carbohydrate 36g
Fiber 2g
Total Fat 3g
Saturated Fat 1g
Cholesterol 63mg
Sodium 1440mg

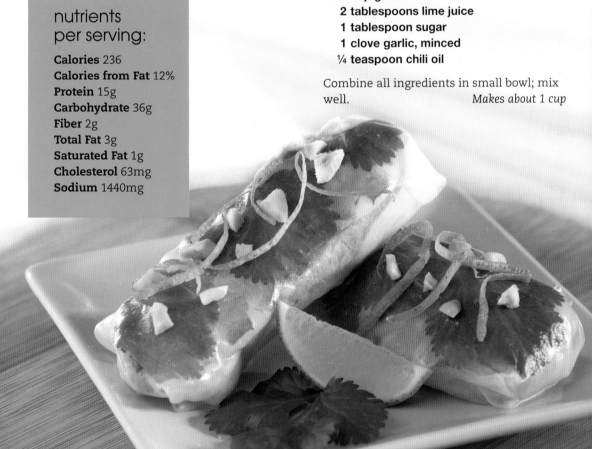

Salmon

Known for its excellent nutrition, firm texture, rich flavor and vivid color, salmon is an ideal fish for eating in place of meat or standard whitefish. Enjoy as a main dish, in a sandwich or salad.

Benefits

Salmon is a great source of protein, but the fatty acids in salmon are what make it a star. You can't find a much healthier fish, especially when it comes to its high omega-3 fat content. These polyunsaturated fats play an important role in almost every aspect of maintaining overall good health, including helping to prevent heart disease and some cancers. And thanks to their positive role in brain development and cognitive function, they may help prevent Alzheimer's disease and depression. Eat salmon or another rich source of omega-3s about twice a week to reap the benefits.

Selection and Storage

Salmon is either wild or farmed, with the majority of it farmed nowadays. Farmed is easier to find and cheaper than wild, but wild is nutritionally better and usually has richer flavor, too. Atlantic salmon is almost all farmed, whereas Pacific (usually Alaskan) salmon is most often wild. Of the pacific species, Chinook, or king, salmon is superior. Fresh salmon is available in fillets or steaks. Keep salmon in the refrigerator for just a couple of days before using, or freeze for longer storage. Salmon is also available canned or in pouches as with tuna, or smoked in a variety of styles.

Preparation

Salmon can be grilled, baked, broiled or steamed. Cook salmon through but be careful not to overcook and dry it out. The skin is edible, although many people choose to remove it for texture.

Recipe Suggestions

Some people prefer to simply season salmon with olive oil, salt and pepper to let its full flavor stand on its own, but it does pair very well with a variety of flavors. Try serving it with a fresh fruit salsa, maple syrup glaze, teriyaki sauce, mustard sauce or creamy dill sauce. Or coat it with ground nuts before cooking for added crunch. Add cooked or canned salmon to any type of green salad, pasta dish or casserole. Or try it in patties as an appetizer, light entrée or in a sandwich.

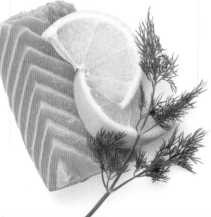

speedy salmon patties

- 1 can (12 ounces) pink salmon, undrained
- 1 egg, lightly beaten
- ¼ cup minced green onions
- 1 tablespoon chopped fresh dill
- 1 clove garlic, minced
- ½ cup rice flour
- 1½ teaspoons baking powder
- Vegetable oil

1. Drain salmon, reserving 2 tablespoons liquid. Place salmon in medium bowl; break apart with fork. Add reserved liquid, egg, green onions, dill and garlic; mix well.

2. Combine rice flour and baking powder in small bowl; add to salmon mixture. Mix well and shape into six patties.

3. Heat oil in large skillet to 350°F. Add salmon patties; cook until golden brown on both sides. Remove from oil; drain on paper towels. Serve warm.

Makes 6 patties (2 patties per serving)

nutrients per serving:

Calories 523
Calories from Fat 60%
Protein 30g
Carbohydrate 23g
Fiber 1g
Total Fat 35g
Saturated Fat 5g
Cholesterol 156mg
Sodium 701mg

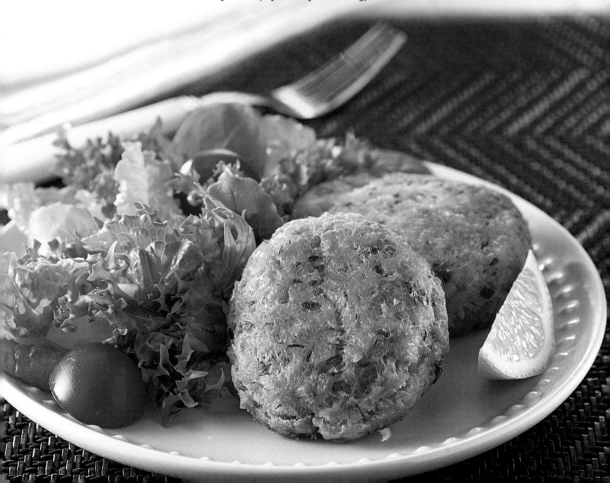

Sesame Seeds

Sesame seeds are a versatile and popular addition in many different cuisines, adding nutrients, a nutty, slightly sweet taste and a delicate crunch and seasoning to dishes.

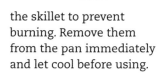

Benefits

For their tiny size, sesame seeds offer many important nutrients. They are rich in many minerals, including copper (an anti-inflammatory), magnesium (for supporting the health of lungs and blood vessels), calcium (for strong bones) and potassium (for healthy blood pressure). Sesame seeds have one of the highest amounts of cholesterol-lowering phytosterols of all the nuts and seeds. They also contain phytonutrients called lignans, which have been shown to help fight some cancers.

Selection and Storage

Sesame seeds are available unhulled, in which they retain a thin, edible shell that can be red, brown or black. More commonly though, sesame seeds are hulled and are tan or beige. They can be found in packages or in the bulk section of the supermarket. Due to their high oil content, sesame seeds are susceptible to rancidity and must be kept in an airtight container at room temperature up to three months or refrigerated up to six months. Sesame oil, made from sesame seeds, is available either plain or toasted and can be found with other oils or in the Asian section of the supermarket.

Preparation

Toast sesame seeds to intensify their flavor before adding them to dishes. Spread them in a dry skillet and toast over medium heat for just a couple of minutes or until they turn light golden brown, shaking the skillet to prevent burning. Remove them from the pan immediately and let cool before using.

Recipe Suggestions

Sesame seeds add a delightful crunch just sprinkled on many dishes, particularly stir-fries and salads. Add them to breads, muffins or cookies for a mild crunchy texture and flavor. They make a great dressing for salads, vegetables or noodles when toasted and mixed with rice vinegar, soy sauce, garlic and ginger. When toasted and combined with sea salt, they make the simple seasoning called gomasio (which is also available in natural food stores). In addition, sesame seeds are the main ingredients in tahini, or sesame seed paste, which is used in many Middle Eastern dishes, including hummus.

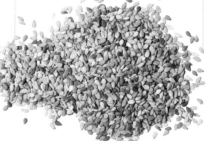

Shellfish

Shellfish is a broad seafood category in which the creature has its skeleton on the outside. It includes crustaceans—including crab, lobster and shrimp—and mollusks—including clams, oysters, mussels and scallops.

Benefits

Shellfish are an excellent source of protein. Compared to other sources of animal protein, shellfish are lower in total fat, including harmful saturated fat, and calories. Shellfish are very good sources of the omega-3 fats that are associated with a lower risk of heart disease and cancer. These beneficial polyunsaturated fats also are important for brain function and may help lower blood pressure and reduce damaging inflammation.

Selection and Storage

It is very important to buy shellfish from a trusted source. Shop for shellfish at your usual grocery store if the selection looks well handled and fresh, and the turnover is frequent. Or go to a specialty seafood shop where there is a wider, often fresher, variety. Most shellfish should be kept alive until ready to cook, except shrimp and scallops. Lobsters and crabs should be active and show leg movement. Oysters, mussels and clams (bivalves) should close their shells when tapped; avoid any with cracked shells. Fresh shellfish should be eaten within two days of purchase. Buying frozen shellfish is an option if you don't plan on eating it very soon. Crabmeat is commonly sold in cans or pouches and can be found in the supermarket with other packaged seafood.

Preparation

Thaw frozen shellfish in the refrigerator completely before cooking, and always keep shellfish cold before you prepare it. Shellfish should be thoroughly cooked, but not overcooked so it doesn't get rubbery and tough. Steam bivalves until the shells open; discard any that don't open. Cook shrimp, scallops and lobster until the flesh turns opaque.

Recipe Suggestions

Fresh lobsters are a treat and best simply boiled and served with melted butter. Fresh crabs are also special and often served like lobster, but crabmeat is much more versatile and can be used in a variety of appetizers and main dishes. Enjoy bivalves on their own in their cooking broth or combined in a seafood stew or added to pasta. Shrimp are extremely versatile and can be served on their own as an appetizer or added to salads, stews or casseroles.

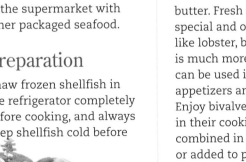

Sorghum Flour

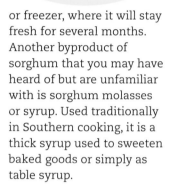

This flour, made from the cereal grass sorghum, is a welcome addition to the gluten-free pantry. Some find the flavor similar to wheat flour, so it makes a great flour substitute in gluten-free baking.

Benefits

Sorghum is somewhat similar to millet, so their flours share comparable health benefits, which are better than many other gluten-free flours. Sorghum flour is one of the more nutritious gluten-free options, being high in protein and insoluble fiber. It also contains a decent amount of antioxidants and iron. It is digested slowly, keeping you fuller for longer.

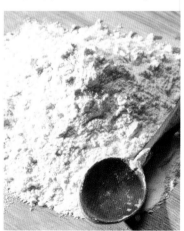

Sorghum flour is beneficial in gluten-free baking because it helps produce foods with a texture more like that of wheat, as opposed to the gumminess that rice flours can cause. While the mild, bland flavor and light color of sorghum flour is best appreciated in gluten-free baking, it can be used in many different dishes, as well.

Selection and Storage

Sorghum flour is more popular in other cuisines, including African and Indian, so it is sometimes referred to with a different name, such as milo or jowar flour. Sorghum flour is most often found among specialty flours in natural food stores, usually near other gluten-free foods, and in ethnic markets. Store it in the refrigerator or freezer, where it will stay fresh for several months. Another byproduct of sorghum that you may have heard of but are unfamiliar with is sorghum molasses or syrup. Used traditionally in Southern cooking, it is a thick syrup used to sweeten baked goods or simply as table syrup.

Preparation

Sorghum flour is included in both flour blends provided in this book, and it is often found in other prepared gluten-free flour blends as well, because of its versatility and the solid nutrition and mild taste it gives baked goods.

Recipe Suggestions

Use sorghum flour in a flour blend in recipes for breads (yeast and quick), breakfast pastries, cookies or cakes. You can also try substituting up to one quarter of sorghum flour for another flour in a recipe.

cinnamon scones

- 2 cups Gluten-Free All-Purpose Flour Blend (page 5)*, plus additional for work surface
- ¼ cup sugar
- 2½ teaspoons baking powder
- ¾ teaspoon salt
- ¾ teaspoon xanthan gum
- ½ teaspoon baking soda
- ⅓ cup cinnamon chips
- ½ cup (1 stick) cold butter, cut into small pieces
- ¾ cup whole milk
- ½ cup plain low-fat yogurt
- 2 tablespoons cinnamon-sugar

*Or use any all-purpose gluten-free flour blend that does not contain xanthan gum.

nutrients per serving:

Calories 216
Calories from Fat 49%
Protein 3g
Carbohydrate 26g
Fiber 1g
Total Fat 12g
Saturated Fat 7g
Cholesterol 22mg
Sodium 382mg

1. Preheat oven to 425°F.

2. Combine 2 cups flour blend, sugar, baking powder, salt, xanthan gum and baking soda in large bowl. Add cinnamon chips; toss to combine. Cut in butter with pastry blender or two knives until coarse crumbs form.

3. Whisk milk and yogurt in small bowl until combined. Gradually add to dry ingredients, stirring just until dough begins to form. (You may not need all of yogurt mixture.)

4. Transfer dough to floured surface. Knead 5 or 6 times until dough holds together.

5. Divide dough into two pieces. Pat each piece into 5-inch circle, about ½ inch thick. Cut each circle into six wedges using floured knife. Place scones 2 inches apart on baking sheet. Sprinkle with cinnamon-sugar.

6. Bake 10 to 14 minutes or until lightly browned. Cool completely on wire rack. *Makes 12 scones*

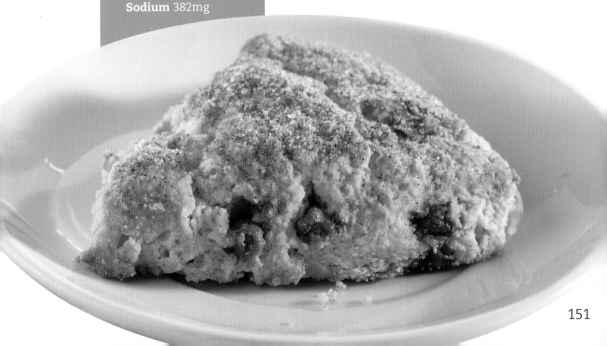

Soybeans

Benefits

Soybeans contain isoflavones, a phytonutrient associated with healthy cholesterol levels that may also help protect against cancer, high blood pressure and osteoporosis. Soybeans provide high-quality protein and a good amount of fiber, both which help fill you up. They also provide essential omega-3 fats that help reduce inflammation and may help lower the risk of cancer and heart disease. Soybeans are lower in carbohydrates than other legumes.

Selection and Storage

Soybeans are available in many different forms, including soy flour, soy milk, soy sauce, soybean oil, soy nuts, tofu, tempeh, dried soybeans and edamame, which are fresh green soybeans. Edamame are a popular snack found in

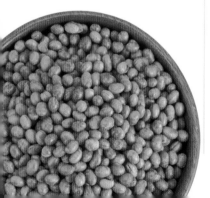

Prized by the Chinese for many thousands of years, soybeans are relatively new to the United States. Used to produce a wide variety of products, soybeans on their own are a versatile and healthy addition to a gluten-free diet.

Japanese restaurants, but they are becoming more popular for use in everyday cooking. Fresh edamame are occasionally available in the produce section of ethnic markets. Frozen edamame are more widely available in large supermarkets, either packaged in the pods or shelled.

Preparation

To cook edamame in the pods, boil them in a large pot of salted water for about 5 minutes. Drain, sprinkle with salt and serve hot or at room temperature in a bowl, with an extra bowl for the discarded pods. To eat them, bite the pods and squeeze out the beans with your teeth (or squeeze the pods with your fingers and press the beans into your mouth), making sure not to eat

the tough pods. The beans should be bright green and crisp-tender. If using shelled edamame, follow the package directions for cooking them, which may include steaming, sautéing or microwaving in addition to boiling. You may enjoy them hot or cold.

Recipe Suggestions

Edamame make a great substitution for other legumes in almost any dish. Add them to your meal if you are going meatless or just want a boost of protein and fiber. Enjoy edamame in the pods as an appetizer or snack, or add them, shelled, to soups, stews, salads, stir-fries and pasta, rice or egg dishes. Puréed shelled edamame make a great dip to serve with fresh veggies and crackers.

edamame hummus

1 package (16 ounces) frozen shelled edamame, thawed
2 green onions, coarsely chopped (about ½ cup)
½ cup loosely packed fresh cilantro
3 to 4 tablespoons water
2 tablespoons canola oil
1½ tablespoons lime juice
1 tablespoon honey
2 cloves garlic
1 teaspoon salt
¼ teaspoon black pepper
Rice crackers, baby carrots, cucumber slices and sugar snap peas

1. Combine edamame, green onions, cilantro, 3 tablespoons water, oil, lime juice, honey, garlic, salt and pepper in food processor; process until smooth. Add additional water to thin dip, if necessary.

2. Serve with rice crackers and vegetables for dipping. Store leftover dip in refrigerator up to four days.

Makes about 2 cups (2 tablespoons per serving)

nutrients per serving:

Calories 55
Calories from Fat 49%
Protein 3g
Carbohydrate 4g
Fiber 2g
Total Fat 3g
Saturated Fat 0g
Cholesterol 0mg
Sodium 148mg

Soy Flour

Ground from roasted soybeans, soy flour is known for having a strong, nutty flavor. Like other soy products, this flour offers a wealth of protein, making it a wise choice when selecting gluten-free flours.

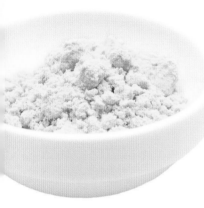

Benefits

More healthful than many other gluten-free flours, soy flour is very high in protein. It is also rich in fiber and the phytonutrients isoflavones. Using soy flour in gluten-free baked goods helps provide a moist, soft texture and preserves freshness. It also imparts a richer flavor and deeper yellow color than most other gluten-free flours. Soy flour is an important ingredient in a slew of commercial foods, from prepared baked goods to processed meat products to frozen foods.

Selection and Storage

Soy flour is most often found among specialty flours in natural food stores, usually near other gluten-free foods. Soy flour comes either full fat (regular), low-fat or defatted. The full fat kind is least commonly available, and it is very perishable and prone to rancidity. The low-fat or defatted kind has had most or all of the oil from the soybeans removed before grinding. Store it in the refrigerator or freezer, where it will stay fresh for several months.

Preparation

Some brands of soy flour toast it, thereby enhancing its flavor. If it has not been toasted already you might try doing so at home. Soy flour is not usually present in prepared gluten-free flour blends, but it can be added to baked goods in small amounts. Because the flavor of soy flour tends to be intense, it is best to use only a small quantity. It is not the best gluten-free flour to use in a recipe for a delicately flavored food. Combining it with other strong flavors, such as chocolate in baking, is an easy way to mask the distinctive beany taste.

Recipe Suggestions

Soy flour's versatility extends its uses beyond just gluten-free baking. Use it as a thickener for gravies and sauces. It can act as an egg substitute when mixed with water. Add it to batter for fried foods to help absorb less fat. You can even use it to make your own soymilk.

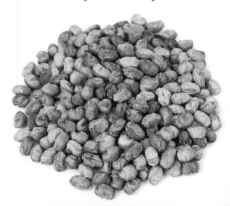

gluten-free brownies

¼ **cup soy flour**
¼ **cup cornstarch**
1 **teaspoon baking soda**
¼ **teaspoon salt**
½ **cup (1 stick) margarine**
1 **cup packed brown sugar**
½ **cup unsweetened cocoa powder**
½ **cup semisweet chocolate chips**
1 **teaspoon vanilla**
2 **eggs**

1. Preheat oven to 350°F. Spray 8-inch square baking pan with nonstick cooking spray. Combine soy flour, cornstarch, baking soda and salt in small bowl.

2. Melt margarine in large saucepan over low heat. Add brown sugar; cook and stir until sugar is completely dissolved. Remove from heat; sift in cocoa and stir until combined. Add flour mixture; stir until smooth. (Mixture will be thick.)

3. Stir in chocolate chips and vanilla. Add eggs; beat until smooth and well blended. Pour batter into prepared pan.

4. Bake 25 to 30 minutes or until toothpick inserted into center comes out almost clean.

Makes 9 brownies

nutrients per serving:

Calories 279
Calories from Fat 44%
Protein 4g
Carbohydrate 37g
Fiber 3g
Total Fat 15g
Saturated Fat 4g
Cholesterol 41mg
Sodium 278mg

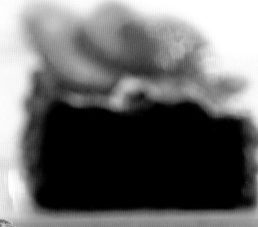

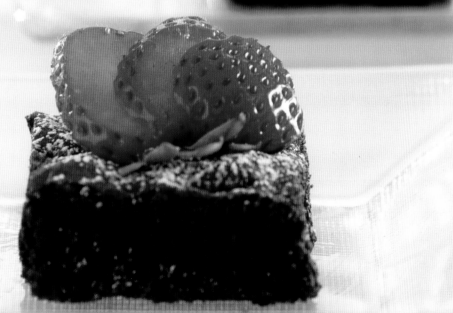

Spaghetti Squash

When raw, spaghetti squash has flesh that is solid like that of other kinds of squash, but when cooked, its flesh separates into spaghetti-like strands, offering a great substitute for gluten-containing pasta.

Benefits

Even though gluten-free pasta is available, usually made from brown rice or quinoa and corn, spaghetti squash is a naturally gluten-free alternative to pasta. It also has the health benefits of being a low-carbohydrate vegetable as opposed to the heavier pastas made from grains. Also unlike gluten-free pasta substitutes, spaghetti squash is very low in calories. It is high in fiber, vitamins A and C, folate and potassium.

Selection and Storage

Being a winter squash, spaghetti squash has a peak season from early fall through winter. It is large and oblong shaped and somewhat resembles a yellow watermelon. Choose bright yellow, hard and smooth spaghetti squash; avoid greenish squash and any with bruised or cracked skin. Store spaghetti squash at room temperature for several weeks.

Preparation

Spaghetti squash must be cooked in order to achieve the spaghetti-like strands. Pierce the whole squash with a knife in several places and bake at 375°F for about an hour or until tender. Let it cool slightly before cutting it in half lengthwise, scooping out the seeds and pulp with a spoon—taking care not to also discard the good flesh underneath—then separating the flesh into strands with a fork. Discard the skin. Or to save time, prepare it in the microwave. Cut the raw squash in half or quarters (you might need to first soften the whole squash in the microwave for a couple minutes) and remove the seeds. Microwave squash pieces for about 8 minutes, let cool slightly, then separate the flesh with a fork.

Recipe Suggestions

Spaghetti squash does not have a strong flavor on its own, so you'll need to dress it up with your favorite toppings. Keep it simple as a side dish by serving it with butter, mixed fresh herbs, salt and black pepper. For a main dish, toss spaghetti squash with chopped cooked fresh vegetables, marinara sauce and Parmesan cheese. Or bake cooked squash in a cheesy gratin or a casserole like you would in any baked pasta recipe.

spaghetti squash alfredo

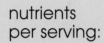

4 cups cooked spaghetti squash (see Note)
½ teaspoon salt
½ teaspoon black pepper
¼ cup (½ stick) butter
1 teaspoon minced garlic
1 cup whipping cream
½ cup grated Parmesan cheese, plus additional for garnish
1 tablespoon olive oil
12 ounces (about 2 cups) frozen cooked shrimp, thawed
Chopped fresh basil (optional)

1. Sprinkle squash with salt and pepper. Melt butter in 12-inch nonstick skillet over medium-high heat. Add garlic; cook 30 seconds. Add squash; cook and stir 2 to 3 minutes or until heated through. Add cream; cook and stir 3 minutes or until sauce begins to thicken. Stir in ½ cup cheese; cook 2 minutes or until cheese is melted. Cover to keep warm; set aside.

2. Meanwhile, heat oil in large nonstick skillet over high heat. Add shrimp; cook and stir until heated through.

3. To serve, top squash mixture with shrimp. Garnish with additional cheese and basil. *Makes 4 servings*

Note: Two medium spaghetti squash (3 to 3½ pounds) will yield about 4 cups cooked squash. Cover and refrigerate any leftover squash for other another use.

nutrients per serving:

Calories 524
Calories from Fat 72%
Protein 24g
Carbohydrate 13g
Fiber 2g
Total Fat 43g
Saturated Fat 24g
Cholesterol 252mg
Sodium 655mg

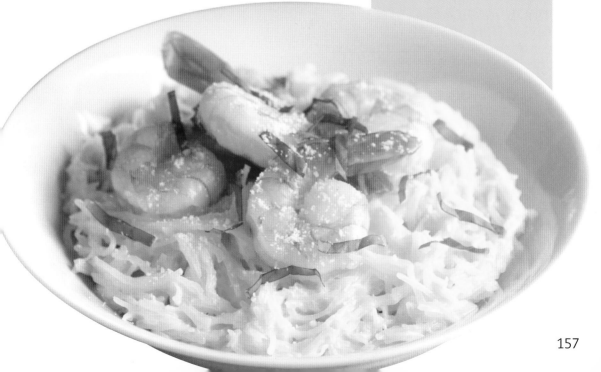

Spices

Whereas herbs come from the leafy part of a plant, spices come from the bark, buds, fruit, roots, seeds or stems of plants. Used for seasoning sweet and savory foods, spices provide a boost of flavor and nutrients to any dish.

Benefits

Spices are widely enjoyed for their warm, unique flavors. Even though we use such small amounts of spices in recipes, we reap a ton of health benefits. Cinnamon has one of the highest antioxidant levels of all the spices, providing the same amount in 1 teaspoon cinnamon as ½ cup of blueberries. Nutmeg, cloves and allspice all have anti-inflammatory properties and help heal digestive woes, which is key for those with gluten intolerance. Turmeric, which is less common on its own but is a main ingredient in

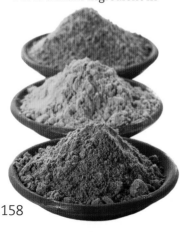

curry powder, has excellent anti-inflammatory and anticancer benefits. It also has been found to offer protection from cardiovascular problems and Alzheimer's disease.

Selection and Storage

Spices are available ground and whole. Ground spices are undoubtedly more convenient, but they lose their aroma and flavor much quicker than whole, so when buying ground, buy it in small quantities. Ground spices will last up to six months. You can buy spices in any supermarket, but for a wider and more interesting variety, you might want to check out specialty spice shops.

Preparation

Spices are occasionally called for in whole form, but they can be easily ground in a small spice or coffee grinder or mortar and pestle. To intensify their flavor before grinding, toast the spices in a dry skillet for 30 seconds or until they release their fragrance. Grind only as much as you need to use in the recipe. Take care when handling ground spices, as many are strongly colored (especially turmeric) and can potentially stain.

Recipe Suggestions

Cinnamon, nutmeg, cloves and allspice are commonly used in winter and holiday baking, especially for quick breads, muffins and cakes. Flavor mulled cider or wine with these spices in whole form for a warm treat. Sprinkle cinnamon over cold and hot cereals, yogurt and even coffee. Make your own curry powder with turmeric for use in Indian-inspired dishes, or add extra to prepared curry powder. Try adding turmeric to brown rice and lentils for a healthy side dish.

Spinach

Of all the healthy leafy greens, spinach is often preferred because it is simple to prepare, has a rich, earthy flavor without too much bitterness and, thanks to Popeye, has a reputation for being "power-packed."

Benefits

Spinach is one of the highest foods in terms of nutrient richness. Loaded with vitamins and minerals, spinach is also one of the best sources of many essential phytonutrients, including carotenoids and flavanoids. These antioxidants have important anti-inflammatory and anticancer properties and also help fight high blood pressure, heart disease, stroke and eye diseases. Spinach is richest in vitamins K, A, C, E and folate; minerals iron, manganese and magnesium; and fiber.

Selection and Storage

Spinach has curly or smooth leaves. The size of leaves range depending on maturity; baby spinach is a variety that is very young with small, tender, mild leaves. Choose spinach with crisp, dark green leaves. Avoid any leaves that are limp and yellowed. Store unwashed spinach in a loose plastic bag in the refrigerator for up to four days. Because they tend to be very gritty, be sure to thoroughly wash leaves just before you use them under cool running water. Prewashed spinach is available in the prepared produce section of the supermarket. Frozen and canned spinach are also readily available.

Preparation

Baby spinach is best for eating raw like in a salad. To sauté spinach for an easy side dish, cook and stir spinach in a skillet with olive oil and garlic just until it wilts, which usually takes a couple minutes. Season with a little lemon juice, salt and pepper. Mature spinach should be boiled briefly. Bring a large pot of water to a rapid boil; boil spinach, uncovered, for 1 minute, then drain and press out all the water. Serve as is with your favorite dressing or add to a variety of dishes.

Recipe Suggestions

Sautéed spinach makes a great side dish. Use raw spinach in place of lettuce in a salad; enjoy it topped with fruit, a crumbled soft cheese, toasted nuts and a sweet vinaigrette. Or add raw spinach to sandwiches or wraps. Add raw or thawed frozen spinach to soups, stews, casseroles or pasta dishes.

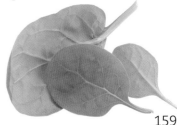

Summer Squash

Unlike winter squash, all parts of summer squash are edible, including the skins and seeds. Summer squash have a tender, delicate and sweet flavor that makes them a tasty addition to a wide variety of dishes year-round.

Benefits

Summer squash are good sources of many important antioxidants, including vitamins C and A and carotenoids. The antioxidants in summer squash are more concentrated in the skins, so it's important to eat the entire squash. (Fortunately, the skins of summer squash are soft and thin, so it's easy to do so.) The high water content of summer squash makes them one of the least caloric vegetables, so along with their decent fiber, summer squash are an excellent filling light vegetable.

Selection and Storage

There are many different types of summer squash, the most common being yellow crookneck and green zucchini. Saucer-shaped pattypan squash is less common but still worth seeking out for a change of pace. As their name suggests, summer squash are best in the summertime, although they are available year-round. Look for squash that are heavy for their size and have smooth, unblemished skins. Summer squash are fragile and need to be stored in the refrigerator for only a few days.

Preparation

One advantage of summer squash is that they can be eaten raw, so when it's hot out and you don't want to cook, you still are able to enjoy them. Simply slice and serve them with your favorite vegetable or bean dip. Or grate them into long, thin strips and use them as a clever substitute for pasta or as a light salad tossed with your favorite dressing. Cooking summer squash can be as simple as sautéing or steaming cut-up squash or grilling thick slices.

Recipe Suggestions

Try a variety of summer squash mixed with eggplant, bell peppers and tomatoes for ratatouille. Add them to risotto, vegetable lasagna, stir-fries or casseroles. Grilled summer squash make a hearty vegetarian sandwich, especially when layered with other grilled veggies, such as eggplant and red bell peppers, cheese and fresh basil leaves. Grated zucchini is a popular addition to many muffins and quick breads, thanks to its natural sweetness. It also gives them moistness and added nutrition, both which are especially important in gluten-free baking.

noodle-free lasagna

- 1 medium eggplant
- 2 medium zucchini
- 2 medium yellow crookneck squash
- 1¼ pounds lean sweet Italian turkey sausage, casings removed
- 2 medium bell peppers, diced
- 2 cups mushrooms, thinly sliced
- 1 can (about 14 ounces) diced tomatoes
- 1 cup gluten-free tomato sauce
- ½ cup coarsely chopped fresh basil
- 1 teaspoon dried oregano
- ½ teaspoon salt
- ¼ teaspoon black pepper
- 1 container (15 ounces) whole-milk ricotta cheese
- 2 cups (8 ounces) shredded mozzarella cheese
- ¼ cup grated Parmesan cheese

1. Preheat oven to 375°F. Cut eggplant, zucchini and yellow squash lengthwise into thin (⅛- to ¼-inch) slices; set aside.

2. Heat large nonstick skillet over medium-high heat. Add sausage; cook 8 to 10 minutes or until cooked through, stirring to break up meat. Drain fat. Transfer to plate.

3. Add bell peppers and mushrooms to skillet; cook and stir 3 to 4 minutes or until vegetables are tender. Return sausage to skillet. Add tomatoes, tomato sauce, basil, oregano, salt and black pepper; cook and stir 1 to 2 minutes or until heated through.

4. Layer one third of eggplant, zucchini and yellow squash in 13×9-inch nonstick baking pan. Spread half of ricotta cheese over vegetables. Top with one third of tomato sauce mixture. Sprinkle evenly with half of mozzarella cheese. Repeat layers once, ending with final layer of vegetables and tomato sauce mixture. Sprinkle with Parmesan cheese; cover with foil.

5. Bake 45 minutes. Remove foil; bake 10 to 15 minutes or until vegetables are tender. Let stand 10 minutes before cutting. *Makes 8 servings*

Tip: To reduce any excess water from eggplant and squash, place sliced vegetables in a colander. Lay a paper towel or clean kitchen towel over the vegetables and weigh them down with a bowl or a couple of cans. Let vegetables drain for 1 to 2 hours before preparing recipe. Or roast the sliced vegetables for 10 minutes in a preheated 350°F oven before preparing recipe.

nutrients per serving:

Calories 443
Calories from Fat 65%
Protein 24g
Carbohydrate 16g
Fiber 5g
Total Fat 34g
Saturated Fat 15g
Cholesterol 88mg
Sodium 1081mg

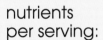

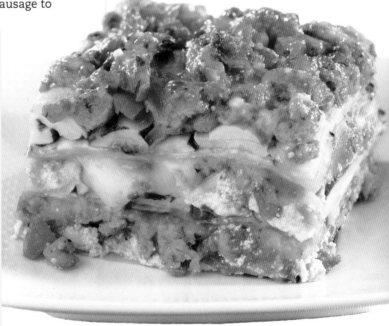

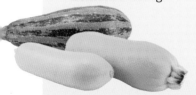

Sweet Potatoes

The sweet potato is a wonderful autumn tuber that should be enjoyed beyond Thanksgiving. One of the oldest vegetables, sweet potatoes have an intensely sweet flavor and are loaded with nutrients.

Benefits

Sweet potatoes are a starchy vegetable loaded with fiber, which helps keep you full. They are especially rich in vitamin A in the form of beta-carotene—which gives sweet potatoes their vibrant orange color—an important antioxidant in fighting chronic diseases as well as inflammation-related conditions. Sweet potatoes also contain a very good amount of infection-fighting vitamin C.

Selection and Storage

Sweet potatoes are not yams, although they are often called that. Yams are a different vegetable, as are regular potatoes. There are many varieties of sweet potatoes. Though the most common is orange, their flesh can range anywhere from white to yellow to pink to purple, and their flavor varies accordingly. Sweet potatoes' peak season is in the fall and early winter, although they are available canned and frozen year-round. Look for fresh sweet potatoes that are firm and unbruised. Store them in a cool, dry, dark place for up to a couple weeks; do not refrigerate them.

Preparation

Sweet potatoes can be prepared in many different ways, and it is important to leave the skin on while cooking to prevent any loss of nutrients. It is best to eat the peel with the flesh, but if you prefer, you can remove the peel after cooking. Boil, bake or microwave whole unpeeled sweet potatoes. Roasting sweet potatoes intensifies their sweetness and provides a subtle crunch on the edge to complement the creamy interior. Chop sweet potatoes into cubes or wedges and toss with olive oil, salt and black pepper. Arrange in a single layer on a baking sheet and bake in a 425°F oven for 30 to 40 minutes.

Recipe Suggestions

Sweet potatoes make excellent side dishes, whether mashed, baked whole or roasted in chunks. Serve them with butter, cinnamon and maple syrup or brown sugar. Mashed cooked sweet potato makes an excellent addition to cakes, quick breads or muffins by adding moisture, sweetness and nutrients. Or try traditional Southern sweet potato pie for a rich dessert and alternative to pumpkin pie.

sweet potato fries

- **1 large sweet potato (about 8 ounces)**
- **2 teaspoons olive oil**
- **¼ teaspoon salt (kosher or sea salt preferred)**
- **¼ teaspoon black pepper**
- **¼ teaspoon ground red pepper**
- **Honey or maple syrup (optional)**

1. Preheat oven to 350°F. Spray baking sheet with nonstick cooking spray.

2. Peel sweet potato; cut lengthwise into long spears. Toss with oil, salt, black pepper and ground red pepper on prepared baking sheet. Arrange sweet potato in single layer (spears should not touch).

3. Bake 45 minutes or until lightly browned. Serve with honey for dipping, if desired.

Makes 2 servings

nutrients per serving:

Calories 139
Calories from Fat 29%
Protein 2g
Carbohydrate 23g
Fiber 4g
Total Fat 5g
Saturated Fat <1g
Cholesterol 0mg
Sodium 301mg

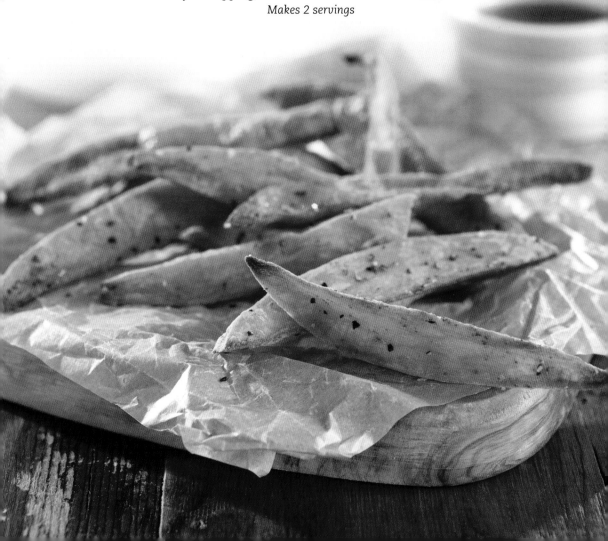

Sweet Rice Flour

Sweet rice flour is sometimes called glutinous rice flour, even though it is gluten-free. It is made from the high-starch short grain rice that is also known as "sticky rice."

Benefits

This flour has a high starch content (it is mostly carbohydrates), though it does contain a small amount of protein. The flavor is milder than the name implies, but it does have a very slightly sweet, milky taste. Used widely in Asian cooking, it is also an excellent thickener and binder that can be used in a variety of gluten-free recipes, particularly sauces and some desserts. It works well when mixed with other gluten-free flours for baking breads, muffins, cakes and cookies because it provides moisture and cohesion.

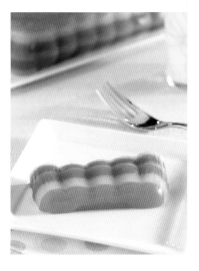

Selection and Storage

In addition to sometimes being labeled as glutinous rice flour, sweet rice flour is often called mochiko, which is the Japanese term, especially in Asian markets. Look for it in the Asian section of large supermarkets, at Asian markets or online. Store it in the refrigerator or freezer, where it will stay fresh for several months.

Preparation

For thickening sauces, mix sweet rice flour with a liquid well to create a smooth, even consistency. Baking recipes that call for sweet rice flour usually only use a small amount, and it is always in conjunction with other flours and sometimes other starches, too.

Recipe Suggestions

Sweet rice flour is especially suited to creating a white sauce, or béchamel, a basic sauce of butter, milk and all-purpose flour, or to be gluten-free, sweet rice flour. This sauce is a key element in dishes such as macaroni and cheese, creamy casseroles and soufflés. Sweet rice flour is the main ingredient for mochi, the traditional Japanese rice cake. Mochi has many applications in Japanese cuisine, such as being made into small sweet confections and added to a variety of soups. Mochi ice cream, which consists of a shell of mochi filled with ice cream, is gaining popularity in the United States in Japanese restaurants and ice cream or yogurt shops.

gf graham crackers

- ½ cup sweet rice flour (mochiko), plus additional for work surface
- ½ cup sorghum flour
- ½ cup packed brown sugar
- ⅓ cup tapioca flour
- ½ teaspoon baking soda
- ½ teaspoon salt
- ¼ cup (½ stick) margarine
- 2 tablespoons plus 2 teaspoons whole milk
- 2 tablespoons honey
- 1 tablespoon vanilla

1. Combine ½ cup sweet rice flour, sorghum flour, brown sugar, tapioca flour, baking soda and salt in food processor; pulse to combine, making sure brown sugar is free of lumps. Add margarine; pulse until coarse crumbs form.

2. Whisk milk, honey and vanilla in small bowl or measuring cup until well blended and honey is dissolved. Pour into flour mixture; process until dough forms. (Dough will be very soft and sticky.)

3. Transfer dough to floured surface; pat into rectangle. Wrap in plastic wrap and refrigerate at least 4 hours or up to 2 days.

4. Preheat oven to 325°F. Cover work surface with parchment paper; generously dust with sweet rice flour.

5. Roll dough to ⅛-inch-thick rectangle on parchment paper using sweet rice-floured rolling pin. (If dough becomes too sticky, return to refrigerator or freezer for several minutes.) Place dough on parchment paper on baking sheet. Score dough into cracker shapes (do not cut all the way through). Prick dough in rows with tines of fork. Place baking sheet in freezer for 5 to 10 minutes or in refrigerator for 15 to 20 minutes.

6. Bake chilled crackers 25 minutes or until firm and lightly darkened. Transfer parchment to wire rack to cool. Cut crackers when cooled slightly.

Makes about 12 crackers
(2 crackers per serving)

Serving Suggestion: Serve crackers as a snack or for S'mores with chocolate and marshmallows.

Tip: Crush extra crackers (or less than perfect ones) and use for graham cracker crumbs.

nutrients per serving:

Calories 264
Calories from Fat 27%
Protein 2g
Carbohydrate 46g
Fiber <1g
Total Fat 8g
Saturated Fat 2g
Cholesterol 1mg
Sodium 398mg

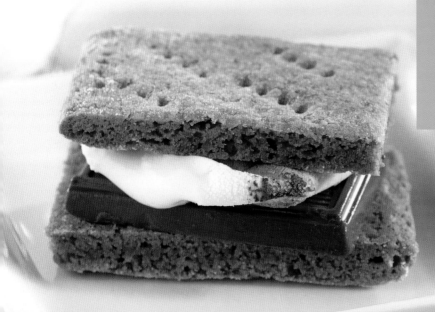

Tapioca

Tapioca is the starch from the tropical cassava plant. Most familiar in pearl form, it is commonly made into tapioca pudding but is also a useful thickener.

Benefits

Tapioca is a staple in many Asian, Indian and South American cuisines, and you will find it most often used in foods from those areas. Americans use instant tapioca to make pudding, but it is also appreciated as a suitable substitute for flour or cornstarch when used as a thickener, much like tapioca flour is. Tapioca is enjoyed for its beadlike texture and chewy bite,

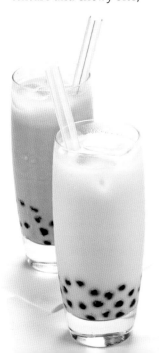

which are softened but mostly retained throughout the cooking process.

Selection and Storage

Tapioca comes in a few different forms, including pearls, flour, granules and flakes. Tapioca pearls, the most commonly used variety, come in several sizes (the largest are more often used in Asian cooking) as well as regular and instant forms. Most people are mainly familiar with the instant kind, also known as quick-cooking, which has been precooked. Instant tapioca is widely available in the baking section of the supermarket, but other varieties should be sought out in specialty ethnic stores. Tapioca can be stored in a sealed container at room temperature indefinitely.

Preparation

Because instant tapioca has already been cooked, it needs little preparation. It is ready to be mixed with other ingredients and briefly cooked according to recipe directions. Regular tapioca needs to be presoaked. For thickening purposes, soak instant tapioca in the liquid called for in the recipe for about 5 minutes before cooking to get the most thickening power. Keep in mind that using instant tapioca will not yield as smooth a result as with tapioca flour, so it's best to use instant when the dish has a chunkier texture to begin with.

Recipe Suggestions

Make tapioca pudding using regular or instant tapioca for a rich and creamy dessert. It is traditionally made with milk, but you can also try a fruit juice of your choice. A more advanced but popular use for large tapioca pearls is for making bubble tea, common in many Asian restaurants.

mixed berry crisp

- 6 cups mixed berries, thawed if frozen
- ¾ cup packed brown sugar, divided
- ¼ cup quick-cooking tapioca
  Juice of ½ lemon
- 1 teaspoon ground cinnamon
- ½ cup rice flour
- 6 tablespoons cold butter, cut into small pieces
- ½ cup sliced almonds

1. Preheat oven to 375°F. Grease 8- or 9-inch square baking pan.

2. Combine berries, ¼ cup brown sugar, tapioca, lemon juice and cinnamon in large bowl. Pour into prepared pan.

3. Combine rice flour, remaining ½ cup brown sugar and butter in food processor; process using on/off pulsing action until mixture resembles coarse crumbs. Add almonds; process using on/off pulsing action until combined. (Leave some large pieces of almonds.)

4. Sprinkle almond mixture over berry mixture. Bake 20 to 30 minutes or until golden brown.

Makes 9 servings

Note: For a gluten-free fruit dessert, a crisp is considerably easier than a pie since you don't need to bother with making a special crust.

nutrients per serving:

Calories 258
Calories from Fat 35%
Protein 2g
Carbohydrate 40g
Fiber 3g
Total Fat 10g
Saturated Fat 5g
Cholesterol 20mg
Sodium 73mg

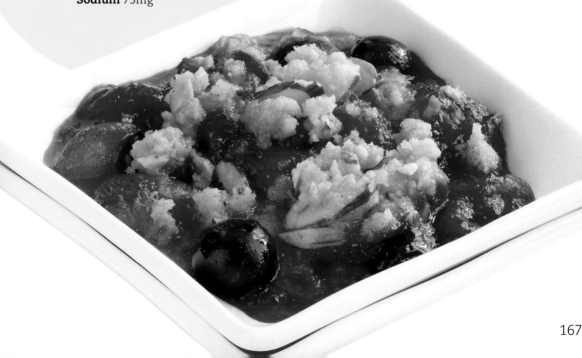

Tapioca Flour

Ground from the cassava root (also called yucca or manioc), tapioca flour, or tapioca starch, is a starchy white flour that has many interesting applications in a gluten-free diet.

Benefits

Popular in many gluten-free flour blends, tapioca starch helps give baked goods a bit of chewiness, a crisp crust and a slightly sweet flavor that is still pretty neutral tasting. Tapioca flour is also good for thickening soups, sauces and especially fruit pie fillings. It is a good substitute for cornstarch in these instances because it thickens at a lower temperature, stays stable when frozen and gives foods a higher gloss. And unlike instant tapioca, the flour dissolves completely, thereby creating a nice smooth texture. Tapioca flour thickens quickly, which is helpful in many instances when you don't have much time, but it also means you need to be careful not to overcook it or it will become stringy.

Selection and Storage

Tapioca flour, also known as tapioca starch, can most often be found among specialty flours in large supermarkets or natural food stores, usually near other gluten-free foods. Store it in the refrigerator or freezer, where it will stay fresh for several months.

Preparation

When using tapioca flour as a thickener, make sure to thoroughly mix it with a liquid before cooking to dissolve it and prevent lumps. For gluten-free baking, tapioca flour is very often a part of flour blends, including both blends in this book. It is also called for in many gluten-free recipes that don't use blends, such as some breads, pancakes, cookies, puddings and even ice creams.

Recipe Suggestions

Use tapioca starch in place of cornstarch as a thickener in any fruit-filled dessert. Try it in combination with other gluten-free flours and starches in recipes for a variety of baked goods. Tapioca flour is the main ingredient in some specific dishes, like Brazilian Cheese Rolls (Pão de Queijo). These moist, chewy rolls are always made with tapioca flour so are gluten-free by nature. They are made of mostly tapioca flour, plus milk, butter, eggs, oil and Parmesan cheese, and are popular in Brazil for breakfast, lunch and dinner.

gluten-free sour cream cranberry coffee cake

Cake

- 2½ cups Gluten-Free All-Purpose Flour Blend (page 5)*
- 2 teaspoons baking powder
- 1½ teaspoons xanthan gum
- 1 teaspoon baking soda
- 1 teaspoon unflavored gelatin
- ½ teaspoon salt
- 1½ cups granulated sugar
- ¾ cup (1½ sticks) butter
- 3 eggs
- 1 cup sour cream
- 2 teaspoons vanilla
- 2 cup fresh or frozen cranberries**

Streusel

- ½ cup packed light brown sugar
- ¼ cup Gluten-Free All-Purpose Flour Blend (page 5)*
- ¾ teaspoon ground cinnamon
- ¼ teaspoon ground nutmeg
- ¼ teaspoon salt
- 3 tablespoons cold butter, cubed

Or use any all-purpose gluten-free flour blend that does not contain xanthan gum.

**If using frozen cranberries, do not thaw before adding them to the batter as they will dye the batter red.*

1. Preheat oven to 350°F. Spray 13×9-inch baking pan with nonstick cooking spray.

2. Combine 2½ cups flour blend, baking powder, xanthan gum, baking soda, gelatin and ½ teaspoon salt in medium bowl.

3. Beat granulated sugar and ¾ cup butter in large bowl with electric mixer at medium-high speed until light and fluffy. Add eggs, one at a time, beating well at medium speed after each addition. Beat in sour cream; scrape side of bowl. Add flour mixture in two additions; beat at low speed until well blended. Beat in vanilla. Fold in cranberries. Pour into prepared pan.

4. Bake 40 minutes. Meanwhile for streusel, combine brown sugar, ¼ cup flour blend, cinnamon, nutmeg and ¼ teaspoon salt in small bowl. Cut in 3 tablespoons butter with pastry blender or two knives until mixture resembles coarse crumbs.

5. Remove coffee cake from oven. Sprinkle evenly with streusel. Bake 10 minutes or until toothpick inserted into center comes out clean. Serve warm or at room temperature.   *Makes 12 servings*

nutrients per serving:

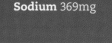

Calories 436	**Total Fat** 22g
Calories from Fat 44%	**Saturated Fat** 12g
Protein 4g	**Cholesterol** 93mg
Carbohydrate 58g	**Sodium** 369mg
Fiber 2g	

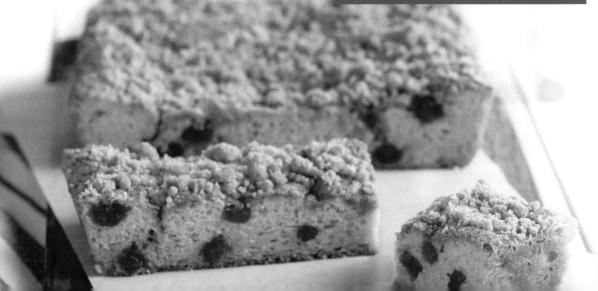

Teff

Teff is the smallest cereal grain in the world that, although a staple in Ethiopia, is relatively unknown in the United States. Both whole teff and teff flour are good nutritious additions to a gluten-free diet.

Benefits

Due to its miniscule size, teff has more of the healthful bran and germ than most other grains. Teff, in both whole and flour forms, is high in protein, fiber, iron and calcium. Whole teff comes in white or red, but the white is nutritionally superior to red. Similar to quinoa and millet, teff has a mild, nutty taste. The flour is used in gluten-free baking for breads, muffins and cookies. Teff flour is most commonly used for making the Ethiopian bread called injera, which is a spongy, fermented flat bread eaten with almost every meal in that country.

Selection and Storage

Teff flour is generally easier to find than whole teff. Look for the flour among specialty flours in natural food stores, usually near other gluten-free foods. Store it in the refrigerator or freezer, where it will stay fresh for several months. Look for whole teff in ethnic markets or order it online.

Preparation

Whole teff can be prepared like most other similar grains, boiled in water or broth until the liquid is absorbed. Teff flour can be added to a gluten-free flour blend or else just combined with other flours in a recipe for bread, muffins or cookies. Try injera at an Ethiopian restaurant if you live near one, but it is not recommended for baking at home because it takes days to prepare.

Recipe Suggestions

Try replacing up to one quarter of another flour with teff flour in a baked good recipe for added variety, nutrition and flavor. Enjoy cooked whole teff alone as a side dish or as a part of a main dish with your favorite vegetables and/or meat. Add it to stir-fries, soups or stews for added body and protein. Or try it as a hot cereal, prepared with juice or milk and garnished with fruit and nuts.

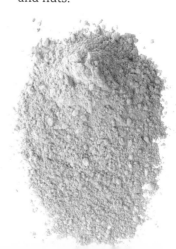

zucchini bread

2½ cups Gluten-Free All-Purpose Flour Blend (page 5)*
⅔ cup packed brown sugar
½ cup teff flour
⅓ cup granulated sugar
1 tablespoon baking powder
2 teaspoons ground cinnamon
1 teaspoon baking soda
1 teaspoon salt
¾ teaspoon xanthan gum
¼ teaspoon ground allspice
¼ teaspoon ground nutmeg
¼ teaspoon ground cardamom
1¼ cups whole milk
2 eggs
¼ cup canola oil
1 teaspoon vanilla
1½ cups grated zucchini, squeezed dry

Or use any all-purpose gluten-free flour blend that does not contain xanthan gum.

1. Preheat oven to 350°F. Grease 9×5-inch loaf pan.

2. Combine flour blend, brown sugar, teff flour, granulated sugar, baking powder, cinnamon, baking soda, salt, xanthan gum, allspice, nutmeg and cardamom in large bowl. Whisk milk, eggs, oil and vanilla in medium bowl.

3. Make well in center of dry ingredients; stir in milk mixture. Stir in zucchini. Pour into prepared pan.

4. Bake 1 hour or until toothpick inserted into center comes out almost clean. Cool in pan on wire rack 5 minutes. Remove to wire rack; cool completely.   *Makes 12 servings*

nutrients per serving:

Calories 264	**Total Fat** 9g
Calories from Fat 30%	**Saturated Fat** 1g
Protein 5g	**Cholesterol** 34mg
Carbohydrate 42g	**Sodium** 450mg
Fiber 2g	

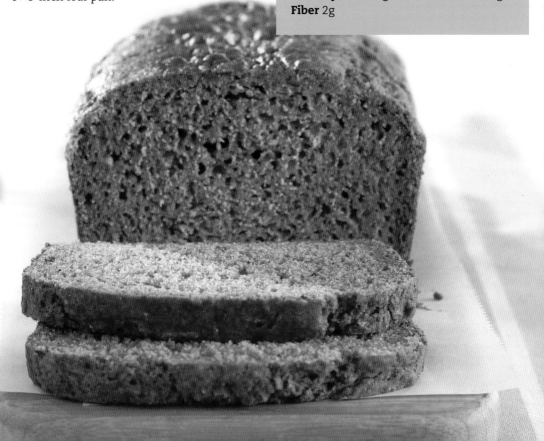

Tomatoes

The applications for tomatoes are endless. Tomatoes, which are actually a fruit but generally considered a vegetable, add a burst of vibrant color, sweet flavor and nutrients to a variety of dishes and cuisines.

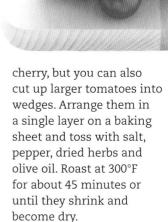

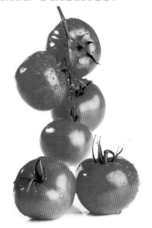

Benefits

Tomatoes are low in calories and high in water and fiber, so they are a great food for those who are trying to watch their weight. Tomatoes are perhaps best known for their high antioxidant content, especially lycopene, which has been found to help reduce the risk of cancer and cardiovascular disease. Lycopene is actually more abundant in cooked tomato products as opposed to fresh tomatoes. Tomatoes have a wealth of vitamin C, which is also an antioxidant and helps supports a healthy immune system.

Selection and Storage

Fresh tomatoes are at their peak in the summer months. Traditionally they are red, but you can also find them orange, pink, yellow, green, even striped. You will find a wonderful variety at your local farmers' market, and the flavors will completely surpass what you are familiar with from supermarket tomatoes. Make sure to store them at room temperature, not in the refrigerator. Canned and jarred tomato products are plentiful in the supermarket, so when out of season, you can still enjoy the benefits of tomatoes.

Preparation

Some people prefer fresh tomatoes as is, but you might want to try roasting them to really concentrate their sweetness. This works best with smaller tomato varieties like grape or cherry, but you can also cut up larger tomatoes into wedges. Arrange them in a single layer on a baking sheet and toss with salt, pepper, dried herbs and olive oil. Roast at 300°F for about 45 minutes or until they shrink and become dry.

Recipe Suggestions

Fresh tomatoes are best sliced in sandwiches or salads or on their own with a sprinkle of salt. If you have an abundance of fresh, you can make your own tomato sauce or salsa, but these products are readily available jarred, and in countless varieties, too. Add a small amount of tomato paste to sauces, soups or stews to add a punch of tomato flavor. Add sun-dried tomatoes to pizza, pasta or casseroles for a tangy, sweet punch.

beef and bean enchiladas

½ **pound ground beef**
1 **can (about 15 ounces) pinto beans, rinsed and drained**
½ **teaspoon ground cumin**
½ **teaspoon salt, divided**
¼ **teaspoon black pepper, divided**
1 **tablespoon canola oil**
1 **onion, chopped**
1 **green bell pepper, chopped**
1 **jalapeño pepper,* minced (optional)**
1 **clove garlic, minced**
1 **can (about 14 ounces) crushed tomatoes**
1½ **teaspoons chili powder**
8 **(5-inch) corn tortillas, softened according to package directions**

*Jalapeño peppers can sting and irritate the skin, so wear rubber gloves when handling peppers and do not touch your eyes.

nutrients per serving:

Calories 480
Calories from Fat 37%
Protein 23g
Carbohydrate 55g
Fiber 15g

Total Fat 20g
Saturated Fat 5g
Cholesterol 33mg
Sodium 891mg

1. Preheat oven to 350°F. Brown beef 6 to 8 minutes in large skillet over medium-high heat, stirring to break up meat. Drain fat.

2. Mash beans in small bowl. Stir beans, cumin, ¼ teaspoon salt and ⅛ teaspoon black pepper into skillet. Remove to plate.

3. Heat oil in same skillet over medium heat. Add onion, bell pepper, jalapeño pepper, if desired, and garlic; cook and stir 8 to 10 minutes or until onion is translucent.

4. Stir tomatoes, chili powder, remaining ¼ teaspoon salt and ⅛ teaspoon black pepper into skillet. Reduce heat to low; simmer 5 minutes.

5. To assemble enchiladas, spoon ¼ cup bean mixture down center of each tortilla. Fold ends to center to enclose filling. Place in 9-inch square baking dish. Top evenly with tomato sauce. Bake 20 minutes.

Makes 4 servings
(2 enchiladas per serving)

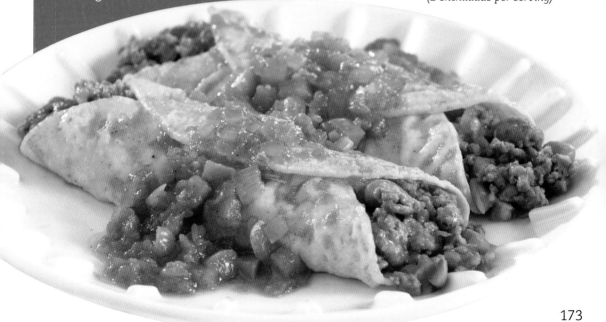

Tuna

Canned tuna is the most popular fish in the United States today, although eating it fresh has been common since ancient times. As convenient as canned is, make sure to try fresh tuna for its dense, meatlike texture and rich flavor.

Benefits

Besides being an excellent source of protein, tuna offers a high amount of the polyunsaturated omega-3 fats that we are recommended to get at least twice a week. Fresh tuna offers even more omega-3s than canned. Omega-3s are very beneficial for the whole body, especially for heart health. Omega-3s are also important in reducing inflammation and may help prevent some cancers.

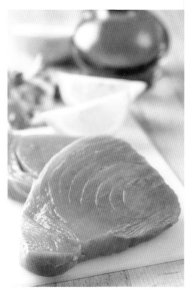

Selection and Storage

The most common varieties of tuna are albacore, which has white flesh and is often called "white," and yellowfin, or ahi, which is deep red in color and labeled "light." Albacore is milder in flavor and pricier than yellowfin. (Bluefin tuna should be avoided due to severe overfishing.) Canned tuna is available packed in water, but you can also find it packed in oil in certain supermarkets. Fresh tuna is usually sold as steaks, but you may also find it in fillets or pieces. Look for it in large supermarkets or at specialty fish markets for the best selection. Refrigerate fresh tuna; use it within one or two days.

Preparation

Fresh tuna can be baked, broiled or grilled. Tuna steaks are best slightly underdone; when cooked all the way through, they lose some of the flavor and texture that makes fresh

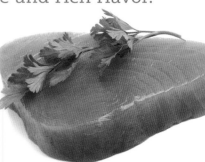

tuna so special. Unlike many other kinds of fish, it is safe for most people to eat undercooked tuna. Many people prefer it rare, with a nice sear on the outside but still pink or red in the middle.

Recipe Suggestions

Fresh tuna does not need a lot of accompaniments. If the tuna is very fresh and of high quality, dressing it in olive oil, salt and pepper is sufficient, but serving it with soy sauce and pickled ginger (as with sushi) is very popular. Tuna salad is the most common use for canned tuna. Try a variation on the typical mayonnaise-based salad by mixing the tuna with fresh lemon juice, olive oil and mustard.

grilled tuna and succotash salad

⅔ cup vegetable oil

¼ cup chopped fresh basil

3 tablespoons balsamic or red wine vinegar

2 tablespoons Dijon mustard

2 tablespoons lemon juice

½ teaspoon salt

½ teaspoon black pepper

4 tuna steaks (about 6 ounces each)

2 cups frozen baby lima beans, cooked according to package directions

1 cup frozen corn, thawed

2 large tomatoes, seeded and chopped

Arugula or spinach leaves

Lemon slices and fresh dill sprigs (optional)

1. Whisk oil, basil, vinegar, mustard, lemon juice, salt and pepper in small bowl.

2. Rinse tuna; pat dry with paper towels. Place tuna in shallow glass dish. Pour ¾ cup oil mixture over tuna; turn to coat evenly. Cover and refrigerate 30 minutes.

3. Prepare grill for direct cooking. Combine lima beans, corn and tomatoes in large bowl. Add remaining oil mixture; toss to coat evenly. Cover and let stand at room temperature until ready to serve.

4. Drain tuna; discard marinade. Grill over medium-high heat 6 to 8 minutes or until desired doneness, turning halfway through grilling time.

5. Arrange arugula on serving plates. Top with tuna. Spoon bean mixture over tuna. Garnish with lemon slices and dill.   *Makes 4 servings*

nutrients per serving:

Calories 806
Calories from Fat 51%
Protein 52g
Carbohydrate 47g
Fiber 12g
Total Fat 45g
Saturated Fat 7g
Cholesterol 64mg
Sodium 546mg

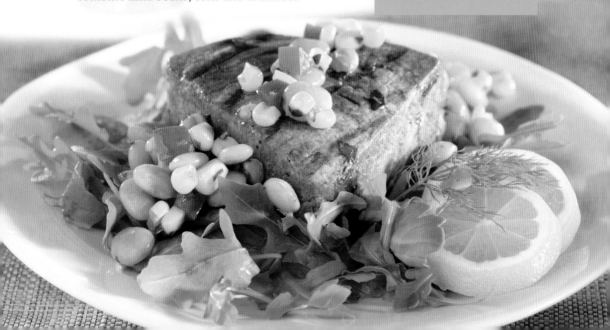

Turkey

Turkey is the star of Thanksgiving, but it shouldn't only be enjoyed then. Due to the increasing emphasis on consuming white rather than red meat, turkey is an excellent protein choice any time of year.

Benefits

Because chicken is so widely consumed, turkey is a refreshing alternative that is similar in flavor, preparation and health benefits. Turkey offers a good amount of protein, B vitamins and various minerals, particularly selenium, and is very low in carbohydrates. As a white meat, turkey is a solid protein choice that is not associated with an increased risk for heart disease and type 2 diabetes like red meat has been has found to be.

Selection and Storage

Turkey is available year-round, fresh and frozen. Fresh birds are recommended because they do not have any preservatives or additives. Buy turkey whole to roast as a centerpiece of a big meal, or in pieces (breasts, drumsticks, cutlets) for simpler, quicker preparation. If possible, select organic turkey—available in large supermarkets, natural food stores and many farmers' markets—for higher-quality meat. Store raw fresh turkey in the refrigerator for up to two days. It can be frozen for longer storage, but keep in mind it takes about one day to thaw 4 to 5 pounds of turkey in the refrigerator. Turkey products, including sausage, bacon and deli meat, are widely available in the supermarket.

Preparation

Purchase and cook turkey with the skin on, even if you plan to remove the skin before eating, because that will help the meat remain moist and flavorful during cooking. Turkey by nature is somewhat dry, so it's important to maintain what moisture there is. Make sure to cook turkey until the internal temperature is 165°F, then let the meat rest for about 10 minutes after it's cooked to seal the juices in.

Recipe Suggestions

Whole turkey is most often roasted—and this might be the most flavorful way of cooking—but you can also bake, grill or even deep-fry it. Prepare turkey cutlets in any way you make chicken cutlets, which have endless possibilities. Substitute ground turkey for ground beef in meat loaves, burgers or chilis. Eat turkey sausage or bacon for breakfast for a lighter meal and a tasty change of pace. Sliced deli turkey makes great sandwiches and even additions to salads.

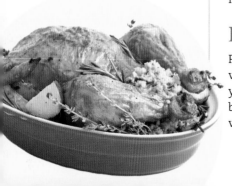

roast turkey breast with sausage and apple stuffing

- **8 ounces bulk pork sausage**
- **1 medium apple, peeled and finely chopped**
- **1 shallot or small onion, finely chopped**
- **1 stalk celery, finely chopped**
- **¼ cup chopped hazelnuts**
- **½ teaspoon rubbed sage, divided**
- **½ teaspoon salt, divided**
- **½ teaspoon black pepper, divided**
- **1 tablespoon butter, softened**
- **1 whole boneless turkey breast (4½ to 5 pounds), thawed if frozen**
- **4 to 6 fresh sage leaves (optional)**
- **1 cup gluten-free chicken broth**

1. Preheat oven to 325°F. Crumble sausage into large skillet. Add apple, shallot and celery; cook and stir over medium-high heat until sausage is cooked through and apple and vegetables are tender. Drain fat.

2. Stir in hazelnuts, ¼ teaspoon each sage, salt and pepper. Spoon mixture into shallow roasting pan.

3. Combine butter and remaining ¼ teaspoon each sage, salt and pepper. Spread over turkey breast. Arrange sage leaves under skin, if desired. Place rack on top of stuffing. Place turkey, skin side down, on rack. Pour broth into pan.

4. Roast 45 minutes. Remove from oven; turn turkey skin side up. Baste with broth. Roast 1 hour or until meat thermometer registers 165°F. Let stand 10 minutes before slicing.

Makes 6 servings

nutrients per serving:

Calories 724
Calories from Fat 51%
Protein 80g
Carbohydrate 6g
Fiber 1g
Total Fat 39g
Saturated Fat 12g
Cholesterol 246mg
Sodium 727mg

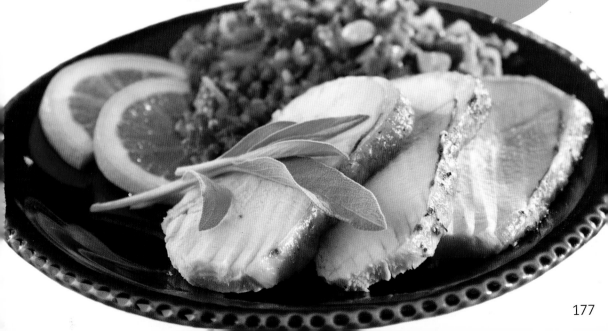

Walnuts

Walnuts are a kind of tree nut, a group of very nutritious nuts. In addition to their health benefits, walnuts add a hearty crunch and distinct, rich flavor to any meal or snack.

Benefits

Walnuts are a health powerhouse. Their high omega-3 fatty acid content is important for heart health and blood pressure regulation. It also benefits brain function and helps fight inflammation. Walnuts are rich in antioxidants, which help improve immune ability and protect the body from damage. Walnuts are even associated with a decreased risk of some cancers. Walnuts have a good amount of protein and fiber, making them an excellent filling snack. Walnuts are also made into fragrant, pleasantly distinctive oil, which provides much of the same nutrition as the nut itself.

Selection and Storage

The most common variety of walnut that is widely available is the English walnut, but there is also the black walnut, which has a more distinct flavor and may be found in some specialty markets. Walnuts are most often already shelled, but you may sometimes also find them in their shells. Shelled walnuts are available in halves, pieces or ground. They can be found in the baking aisle, the snack aisle and in bulk bins. Because of their high fat content, shelled walnuts are prone to rancidity and should be stored in the refrigerator for up to six months. Look for walnut oil with other specialty oils in large supermarkets or natural food stores.

Preparation

In addition to making a wonderful snack on their own, walnuts can be added to a wide variety of both sweet and savory dishes for taste and crunch. As with other nuts, walnuts' flavor is intensified when they are toasted. Arrange walnuts in a single layer on a baking sheet and bake at 350°F for 5 to 7 minutes or until they become fragrant and lightly browned, stirring occasionally.

Recipe Suggestions

Sprinkle chopped walnuts over hot or cold cereals or yogurt for a morning meal or snack. Add them to salads, vegetable dishes or stuffing. Include them in baked goods such as cookies, muffins and quick breads. Mix them into trail mix or make homemade granola using gluten-free oats, dried fruits, honey and chopped walnuts.

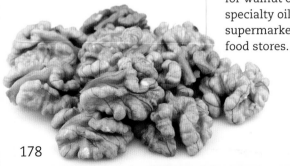

gluten-free thumbprint cookies

- **1 cup (2 sticks) butter, softened**
- **½ cup packed dark brown sugar**
- **2 egg yolks**
- **2 teaspoons vanilla**
- **2 cups Gluten-Free All-Purpose Flour Blend (page 5)***
- **½ teaspoon salt**
- **2 egg whites, beaten**
- **2¼ cups chopped walnuts**
- **¼ cup raspberry jam**

Or use any all-purpose gluten-free flour blend that does not contain xanthan gum.

1. Preheat oven to 375°F. Line baking sheets with parchment paper.

2. Beat butter and brown sugar in large bowl with electric mixer at medium-high speed 2 minutes or until light and fluffy. Add egg yolks and vanilla; beat at low speed, scraping side of bowl, if necessary. Beat in flour blend and salt just until combined.

3. Place egg whites in shallow dish. Place walnuts in separate shallow dish. Roll dough into tablespoonful-size balls. Dip balls into egg whites; roll in walnuts. Place on prepared baking sheets.

4. Using back of small spoon or thumb, make small indent in center of each ball; fill with jam.

5. Bake 12 to 15 minutes or until golden brown and filling is set, rotating sheets halfway through baking time. Cool on baking sheets 5 minutes. Remove to wire racks; cool completely.   *Makes 2 dozen cookies (1 cookie per serving)*

nutrients per serving:

Calories 215	**Total Fat** 16g
Calories from Fat 66%	**Saturated Fat** 6g
Protein 3g	**Cholesterol** 36mg
Carbohydrate 16g	**Sodium** 124mg
Fiber 1g	

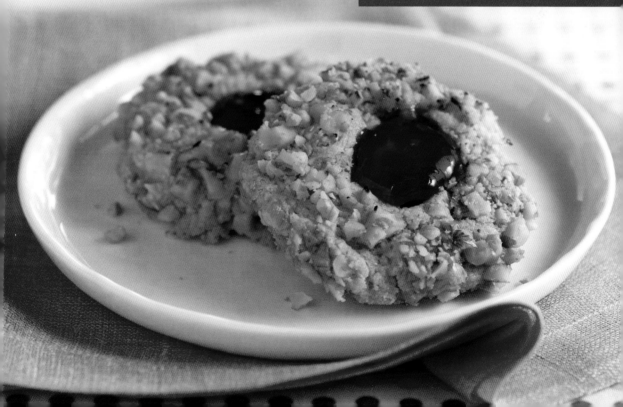

White Rice Flour

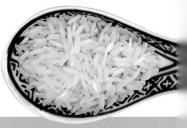

White rice flour is produced from rice that has been hulled to remove the bran and germ and then polished to a powder. It is one of the most commonly used gluten-free flours, especially in baking.

Benefits

Because it is not whole grain, white rice flour is less healthful than brown rice flour and many other gluten-free flours. It contains a small amount of protein and fiber but is much lower in most important nutrients than brown rice flour. Both rice flours are most often interchangeable, but white rice flour is preferred in many gluten-free baking recipes because it does not offer any discernible flavor and it helps make a light, spongy product. Besides its prevalence in gluten-free baking, white rice flour is most commonly used to make a variety of Asian noodles.

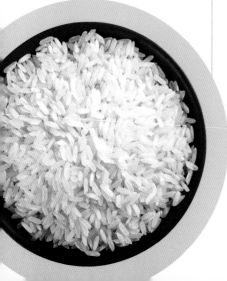

Selection and Storage

White rice flour is most often found among specialty flours in natural food stores, usually near other gluten-free foods. The texture of white rice flour can be slightly gritty, and brands vary in the coarseness of the flour, so you might want to buy different brands at once and compare the textures. Store it in the refrigerator or freezer, where it will stay fresh for several months.

Preparation

Because of the slight coarseness of white rice flour, it's best to use it in combination with other gluten-free flours. It is very often found in many gluten-free bread blends, including the all-purpose blend in this book, because it is so versatile. A blend including white rice flour is good for baking cookies, bars, cakes, muffins, pancakes, crêpes and quick breads, but not yeast breads.

Recipe Suggestions

White rice flour (as well as brown rice flour) is an excellent one-to-one substitute for all-purpose flour when called for in a small amount (up to a couple tablespoons), so you can feel confident when making the switch in non-gluten-free recipes like those. Other applications for white rice flour include thickening casseroles, sauces, gravies and puddings, much as you would also use a small amount of all-purpose flour for.

green bean casserole with homemade french fried onions

3 cups water
1 pound fresh green beans, cut into 2-inch pieces
1 tablespoon vegetable oil
8 ounces cremini mushrooms, chopped
3 tablespoons butter
3 tablespoons rice flour
1 teaspoon salt
¼ teaspoon red pepper flakes
1 cup gluten-free mushroom or vegetable broth
1 cup whole milk
Homemade French Fried Onions (recipe follows)

1. Preheat oven to 350°F. Spray 13×9-inch baking dish with nonstick cooking spray.

2. Bring water to a boil in medium saucepan. Add green beans; cook 4 minutes. Drain.

3. Heat oil in large saucepan or Dutch oven over medium heat. Add mushrooms; cook and stir 8 minutes. Add butter; cook and stir until melted. Stir in rice flour, salt and red pepper flakes. Slowly stir in broth and milk; cook until thickened. Remove from heat. Stir in green beans. Pour into prepared dish.

4. Bake 30 minutes. Meanwhile, prepare Homemade French Fried Onions.

5. Remove casserole from oven. Top with Homemade French Fried Onions. Bake 5 minutes. *Makes 6 to 8 servings*

homemade french fried onions

2 small onions, sliced into rings
½ cup whole milk
½ cup rice flour
½ cup cornmeal
1 teaspoon salt
½ teaspoon black pepper
Vegetable oil

1. Line baking sheet with paper towels. Separate onion rings and spread in shallow dish. Pour milk over onions; toss to coat.

2. Combine rice flour, cornmeal, salt and pepper in large resealable food storage bag; mix well.

3. Heat oil in large heavy skillet over medium-high heat until temperature registers 300°F to 325°F on deep-fry thermometer.

4. Working in batches, add onion rings to food storage bag; shake to coat. Add onions to oil; fry 2 minutes per side or until golden brown. Remove to prepared baking sheet using slotted spoon. Repeat with remaining onions.

Makes about 1½ cups

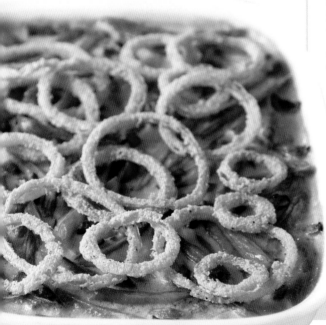

nutrients per serving:

Calories 346
Calories from Fat 51%
Protein 8g
Carbohydrate 36g
Fiber 5g

Total Fat 20g
Saturated Fat 6g
Cholesterol 21mg
Sodium 968mg

Wild Rice

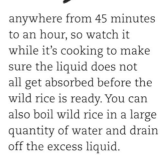

Also called Indian Rice, nutty, chewy and naturally gluten-free wild rice is actually a long grain marsh grass, not rice, traditionally grown in lakes and rivers in the Great Lakes region of the United States.

Benefits

Nutritionally, wild rice is comparable to other whole grains, offering protein, fiber, many minerals, including iron, and some vitamins. Wild rice is an excellent alternative to more common grains you are already familiar with, and it also works very well in a blend of different kinds of rice or grains. It is often more satisfying than brown rice because it is higher in protein, and its chewier, heartier texture and nutty flavor make it a great side dish or stuffing.

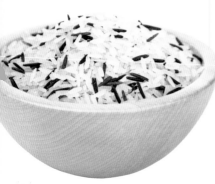

Selection and Storage

Wild rice is not as common as white or brown rice, and it is also more expensive. Wild rice can be found in packages in large supermarkets or natural food stores along with other grains. Often it is sold as a blend with long grain rice or another complementary grain. Store it in a sealed container in a cool, dry, dark place.

Preparation

Rinse wild rice well before preparing it. Cook it in a saucepan on the stovetop as you would other long grain rice, but use a ratio closer to one part wild rice to three parts water or broth. The length of cooking time is more variable, as it depends on the grains of the particular wild rice you are using. It can take anywhere from 45 minutes to an hour, so watch it while it's cooking to make sure the liquid does not all get absorbed before the wild rice is ready. You can also boil wild rice in a large quantity of water and drain off the excess liquid.

Recipe Suggestions

Wild rice is just as versatile as other varieties of rice, so you can easily incorporate it into your favorite rice dishes in place of white or brown rice. It works well as a pilaf with herbs, spices and vegetables of your choice. You can bake it in a casserole, make it into a soup or add it cooked to a salad. It pairs nicely with dried fruits and nuts, as well as mushrooms.

wild rice casserole

1 cup uncooked wild rice
1 large onion, chopped
1 cup (4 ounces) shredded Cheddar cheese
1 cup chopped mushrooms
1 cup chopped black olives
1 cup drained canned diced tomatoes
1 cup tomato juice
⅓ cup vegetable oil
Salt and black pepper

1. Preheat oven to 350°F.

2. Combine rice, onion, cheese, mushrooms, olives, tomatoes, tomato juice and oil in large bowl. Transfer rice mixture to 2½- to 3-quart casserole. Season with salt and pepper.

3. Cover and bake 1½ hours or until rice is tender.

Makes 6 servings

Note: This tastes even better reheated the next day.

nutrients per serving:

Calories 330
Calories from Fat 56%
Protein 10g
Carbohydrate 27g
Fiber 3g
Total Fat 21g
Saturated Fat 6g
Cholesterol 20mg
Sodium 457mg

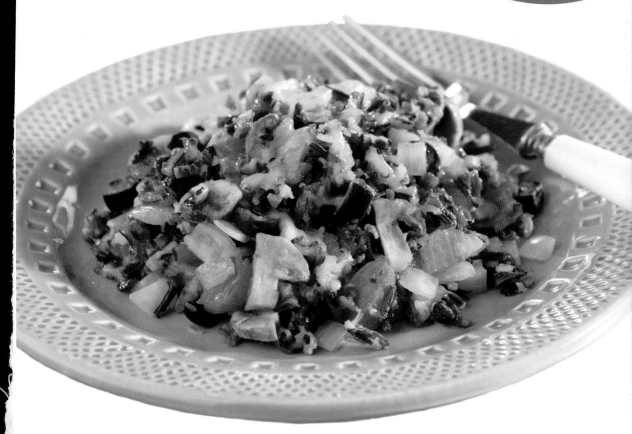

Yeast

Baker's yeast is gluten-free, but whether you're baking with or without gluten, yeast is a necessary ingredient to make breads rise and give them the proper texture.

Benefits

For gluten-free purposes, yeast is most important as a leavening agent in baking gluten-free breads. Yeast is a living organism that produces carbon dioxide and alcohol, which is what helps yeast breads rise. Another type of yeast is nutritional yeast, which may or may not be gluten-free depending on the brand, and it is used as a supplement in many vegetarian or vegan diets.

Selection and Storage

There are two kinds of baker's yeast available, fresh yeast and dry yeast. Fresh is not nearly as common as dry, and most recipes use dry for its convenience. Fresh comes in refrigerated small cakes and only lasts a week or two. Dry yeast comes granulated in small envelopes that can be found in the baking section of the supermarket.

Dry yeast is either active dry or rapid-rise. They can be used interchangeably in most cases, but using active dry yields better flavor and texture.

Preparation

Yeast feeds off of moisture, warmth and food, which is why you combine yeast with a warm liquid and a sweetener to activate it before using in recipes. After it's activated and combined with the remaining ingredients, you knead the dough to introduce air into it. Then, yeast begins the process

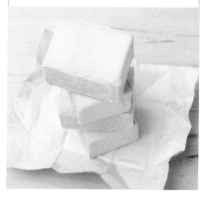

of fermenting and rising the dough when you let the dough rest in a warm place. When doubled in size, bake the bread as is or else punch the dough down, reshape the dough and let it rise a second time before baking, depending on the recipe and type of yeast you are using.

Recipe Suggestions

Yeast is used in recipes for many loaf breads such as sandwich bread, pizza dough and flat breads such as focaccia. Although it is possible to convert recipes for quick breads containing wheat to gluten-free versions with some simple experimentation, yeast breads are trickier and are not recommended for converting. It is best to use recipes already using gluten-free flours in this case.

gluten-free chocolate cherry bread

⅔ cup plus ¼ cup warm water (110°F), divided
1 package (¼ ounce) active dry yeast
3 tablespoons sugar, divided
2 cups Gluten-Free All-Purpose Flour Blend (page 5)*
1½ teaspoons xanthan gum
½ teaspoon salt
5 tablespoons butter, melted and cooled
3 eggs, at room temperature
¾ cup dried sour cherries**
4 ounces bittersweet chocolate, chopped

*Or use any all-purpose gluten-free flour blend that does not contain xanthan gum.

**If dried sour cherries aren't available, you may substitute with other dried cherries or even dried cranberries.

1. Spray 9×5-inch loaf pan with nonstick cooking spray. Combine ¼ cup water, yeast and 1 tablespoon sugar in large bowl; let stand 10 minutes or until foamy.

2. Add flour blend, remaining 2 tablespoons sugar, xanthan gum and salt to yeast mixture. Whisk butter, remaining ⅔ cup water and eggs in small bowl. Gradually beat into flour mixture with electric mixer at low speed until well blended. Scrape side of bowl; beat at medium-high speed 3 minutes or until well blended. Add cherries and chocolate; beat at low speed just until incorporated.

3. Pour batter into prepared pan. Cover; let rise in warm place about 1 hour or until batter almost reaches top of pan.

4. Preheat oven to 350°F.

5. Bake 35 to 40 minutes or until toothpick inserted into center comes out clean. Cool in pan on wire rack 10 minutes. Remove to wire rack; cool completely.   *Makes 12 servings*

Note: This bread may fall slightly after coming out of the oven.

nutrients per serving:

Calories 237
Calories from Fat 41%
Protein 4g
Carbohydrate 33g
Fiber 2g
Total Fat 11g
Saturated Fat 5g
Cholesterol 59mg
Sodium 120mg

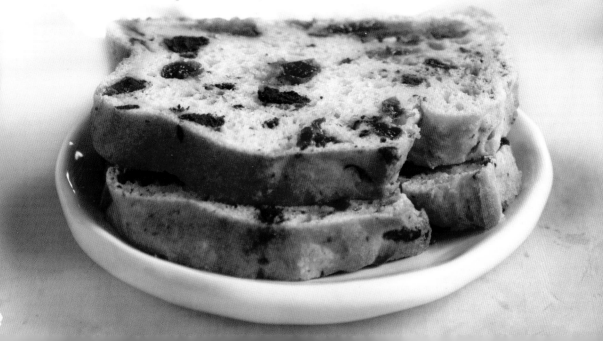

Yogurt

Yogurt has been around for thousands of years and was originally made as a way to preserve milk. Fermenting milk with friendly bacteria results in this beloved creamy, mildly tart treat.

Benefits

Like the milk it is made from, yogurt is high in calcium, which is especially beneficial for bone health. Greek yogurt—yogurt that has been strained to remove much of the liquid whey, lactose and sugar, and as a result is thicker and creamier—is richer in protein and lower in carbohydrates than regular yogurt. With any strained yogurt like Greek, even the nonfat variety maintains a pleasantly rich texture, so you save on fat and calories. Perhaps most importantly, especially for those who are gluten intolerant, yogurt contains live active cultures, which are extremely beneficial for overall health but specifically for easing digestive problems. In gluten-free baking, yogurt helps add moisture and tenderness to breads.

Selection and Storage

The refrigerated yogurt section in the supermarket is bigger and offers more choice than ever before, so you are bound to encounter almost any variety and flavor imaginable. Be sure to check the labels of flavored varieties to be sure they are free of gluten. Due to Greek yogurt's increasing popularity, there are many new brands and flavors now available. New to the market and similar to Greek yogurt because it is also strained, is Icelandic yogurt, or skyr. Although the majority of yogurt is made from cow's milk, it is also available in goat's milk, water buffalo's milk and even vegan varieties in larger or specialty supermarkets.

Preparation

Yogurt's unique taste and texture are best appreciated eaten alone as a snack or as part of a meal. Although there are numerous flavors of yogurt available and convenient, many of these are loaded with added sugars, especially varieties that are aimed towards kids. A simple way to avoid many unwanted additives and to ensure it is gluten-free is to buy plain yogurt and add flavorings yourself.

Recipe Suggestions

For breakfast or a midmorning snack, dress yogurt up with your favorite fruit, nuts and a drizzle of honey. Add yogurt to a fruit smoothie or use it to top hot cereals. Substitute sour cream or mayonnaise with yogurt in creamy dips and salad dressings. The possibilities are endless!

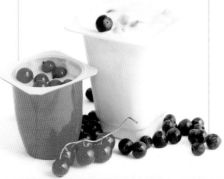

gluten-free waffles

2 eggs
½ cup plain low-fat yogurt
½ cup whole milk
1 cup Gluten-Free All-Purpose Flour Blend (page 5)*
1 tablespoon sugar
1 teaspoon baking powder
1 teaspoon baking soda
½ teaspoon salt
2 tablespoons butter, melted
    Maple syrup and additional butter

*Or use any all-purpose gluten-free flour blend that does not contain xanthan gum.

1. Preheat waffle iron according to manufacturer's directions.

2. Beat eggs in large bowl until light and fluffy. Whisk in yogurt and milk.

3. Combine flour blend, sugar, baking powder, baking soda and salt in medium bowl. Gradually whisk yogurt mixture into flour mixture until smooth. Whisk in 2 tablespoons butter.

4. Add batter to waffle iron by ½ cupfuls for 6-inch waffles (or adjust amount depending on waffle iron). Bake until crisp and browned. Serve with maple syrup and additional butter.

Makes 5 waffles (1 waffle per serving)

Note: Refrigerate or freeze leftover waffles; reheat in toaster oven until crisp.

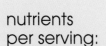

nutrients per serving:

Calories 209
Calories from Fat 43%
Protein 6g
Carbohydrate 24g
Fiber 1g
Total Fat 10g
Saturated Fat 4g
Cholesterol 91mg
Sodium 679mg

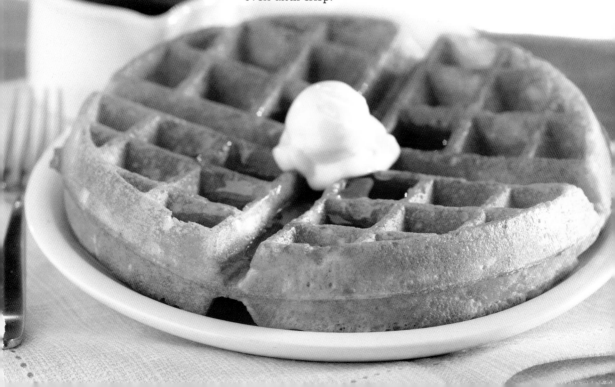

Index

METRIC CONVERSION CHART

VOLUME MEASUREMENTS (dry)

$^1/_8$ teaspoon = 0.5 mL
$^1/_4$ teaspoon = 1 mL
$^1/_2$ teaspoon = 2 mL
$^3/_4$ teaspoon = 4 mL
1 teaspoon = 5 mL
1 tablespoon = 15 mL
2 tablespoons = 30 mL
$^1/_4$ cup = 60 mL
$^1/_3$ cup = 75 mL
$^1/_2$ cup = 125 mL
$^2/_3$ cup = 150 mL
$^3/_4$ cup = 175 mL
1 cup = 250 mL
2 cups = 1 pint = 500 mL
3 cups = 750 mL
4 cups = 1 quart = 1 L

VOLUME MEASUREMENTS (fluid)

1 fluid ounce (2 tablespoons) = 30 mL
4 fluid ounces ($^1/_2$ cup) = 125 mL
8 fluid ounces (1 cup) = 250 mL
12 fluid ounces (1$^1/_2$ cups) = 375 mL
16 fluid ounces (2 cups) = 500 mL

WEIGHTS (mass)

$^1/_2$ ounce = 15 g
1 ounce = 30 g
3 ounces = 90 g
4 ounces = 120 g
8 ounces = 225 g
10 ounces = 285 g
12 ounces = 360 g
16 ounces = 1 pound = 450 g

DIMENSIONS

$^1/_{16}$ inch = 2 mm
$^1/_8$ inch = 3 mm
$^1/_4$ inch = 6 mm
$^1/_2$ inch = 1.5 cm
$^3/_4$ inch = 2 cm
1 inch = 2.5 cm

OVEN TEMPERATURES

250°F = 120°C
275°F = 140°C
300°F = 150°C
325°F = 160°C
350°F = 180°C
375°F = 190°C
400°F = 200°C
425°F = 220°C
450°F = 230°C

BAKING PAN SIZES

Utensil	Size in Inches/Quarts	Metric Volume	Size in Centimeters
Baking or Cake Pan (square or rectangular)	8×8×2	2 L	20×20×5
	9×9×2	2.5 L	23×23×5
	12×8×2	3 L	30×20×5
	13×9×2	3.5 L	33×23×5
Loaf Pan	8×4×3	1.5 L	20×10×7
	9×5×3	2 L	23×13×7
Round Layer Cake Pan	8×1½	1.2 L	20×4
	9×1½	1.5 L	23×4
Pie Plate	8×1¼	750 mL	20×3
	9×1¼	1 L	23×3
Baking Dish or Casserole	1 quart	1 L	—
	1½ quart	1.5 L	—
	2 quart	2 L	—